1993

ETHICAL CONFLICTS IN THE MANAGEMENT OF HOME CARE
The Case Manager's Dilemma

ETHICAL CONFLICTS IN THE MANAGEMENT OF HOME CARE
The Case Manager's Dilemma

Rosalie A. Kane
Arthur L. Caplan
Editors

SPRINGER PUBLISHING COMPANY
New York

Springer Publishing Company, Inc.
536 Broadway
New York, NY 10012

93 94 95 96 97 / 5 4 3 2 1

Library of Congress Cataloging-in-Publication Data

Ethical conflicts in the management of home care: the case manager's dilemma /
    Rosalie A. Kane, Arthur L. Caplan, editors.
        p.   cm.
        Includes bibliographical references and index.
        ISBN 0-8261-8220-8
        1. Aged—Home care—United States—Moral and ethical aspects—case studies.
    2. Aged—Long-term care—United States—Moral and ethical aspects—Case
    studies. 3. Handicapped—Home care—United States—Moral and ethical
    aspects—Case studies. 4. Handicapped—Long-term care—United States—Moral
    and ethical aspects—Case studies. 5. Medical social work—United States—
    Management—Moral and ethical aspects. 6. Social case work—United States—
    Management—Moral and ethical aspects. I. Kane, Rosalie A. II. Caplan, Arthur L.
    RA564.8.E93 1992
    174.2—dc20   92-33131
                                                                                CIP

Printed in the United States of America

The publisher acknowledges the following permissions for material used in Chapter 6:

"The Hunchback in the Park" by Dylan Thomas, from *Poems of Dylan Thomas*.
Copyright © 1943 by New Directions Publishing Corporation. Reprinted by permission
of New Directions Publishing Corp.

Tell Me a Riddle by Tillie Olsen. Copyright © 1956, 1957, 1960, 1961 by Tillie Olsen.
Used by permission of Delacorte Press/Seymour Lawrence, a division of Bantam
Doubleday Dell Publishing Group, Inc.

CONTENTS

Preface and Acknowledgments

The idea for this book grew from the work of the University of Minnesota National Long-Term Care Decisions Resource Center, established in 1988 by a grant from the Administration on Aging. In that capacity, we have frequent contact with state and community programs for the elderly. These programs invariably have a case-management component, and the case managers are frequently troubled by ethical issues. This project represents the ongoing collaboration between the Long-Term Care Decisions Resource Center, which is part of the Institute for Health Services Research in the School of Public Health, and the Center for Biomedical Ethics, to identify and understand ethical issues in long-term care.

Following a format that proved successful in an earlier project (resulting in a 1990 Springer book, *Everyday Ethics: Resolving Dilemmas in Nursing Home Life*), we invited ethicists to prepare written commentaries on cases derived from our empirical study of case managers. We then held a spirited working conference in July 1991, when the draft commentaries were held up to the scrutiny of other philosophers and ethicists as well as researchers and administrators of large case-management programs. The case commentaries and additional reactions from the field were refined in the crucible of that conference.

A project like this is indebted to many people. For the empirical study, summarized in Chapter 2, Colleen King supervised the telephone interviews with case managers; Janis Dehler, Julie Frost, Lana Herskovitz, Tim Jorrisen, and Diane Matson conducted the interviews. Cheryl King Thomas arranged the many details of the working conference. Gloria Kittlesen typed and retyped this manuscript, including the painstaking final version for the typesetter. We are also grateful to the Administration on Aging for its support of the Long-Term Care Decisions Resource Center, and to Brian Hofland and The Retirement Research Foundation for its support of our work on how case managers assess values and preferences. Finally, we appreciate the willingness of our contributors to ply their ethical reasoning and insights to this emerging field, and the willingness of so many case managers and case-management programs to join in the exploration. The comments of the state officials contributing to this book are their own and do not reflect official policy.

Our attention to the ethics of case management commonly evokes a somewhat surprised response. Bioethicists tend to be startled that case managers are so ubiquitous and that they seem so entangled in the important life decisions of disabled older people. Who are these case managers, and how did they get to be important? What is their legal and statutory authority? What is their expertise? These kinds of questions abounded at our 1991 conference on these cases. There is no ancient Hippocratic oath for case managers and no uniform code of ethics. Case managers, whether they be nurses or social workers or have some other training, function in a gray area between health care and social services. They have crept up on bioethicists unaware.

Ethicists must examine the difficult roles of case managers and others who arrange and allocate services for the disabled, often within resource restraints. They should continue to explore the dilemmas of those who are charged to promote the autonomy of their clients and protect them as well, and who must do so with the knowledge that their predictions are imperfect and public opinion often unforgiving. We hope that this book is a first step in what becomes a sustained examination.

ROSALIE A. KANE
ARTHUR L. CAPLAN

PART **I**

INTRODUCTION

Chapter 1

WHAT IS CASE MANAGEMENT, AND WHY DOES IT RAISE ETHICAL ISSUES?

Rosalie A. Kane and Cheryl King Thomas

Case management, sometimes called care coordination, is almost an essential aspect of long-term care for frail elderly and disabled adults. Although definitions vary somewhat, case management is widely perceived as a service function that provides expert assessment of multidimensional needs and assists clients in obtaining needed care. Case management is also increasingly an administrative function; in many programs, case managers allocate or purchase services, they monitor the quality of the services they arrange, and they count their public costs.

By fairly widespread agreement, the functions of a case manager include case finding; comprehensive, structured multidimensional assessment; care planning; implementation of the plan (often with purchase of service); monitoring of the quality of services and the well-being of the client; and reassessment at regular intervals (or on demand) to begin the cycle again. If being ethical supposes being competent and meeting specified minimum standards, case management carries too much ambiguity for easy meeting of this expectation. Developing fixed standards and codifying them into law would be premature. But, as a result of the lack of standardization, there is enormous variation in the training, case-load size, and general modus operandi of case managers.

Case managers tend to work within finite resources, often with fixed budgets. They are asked to give with one hand—that is, to discover a need for services and help clients get the necessary services. They are asked to hold back with the other hand—that is, to be parsimonious, to get by with as little expenditure as possible, and to encourage as much volunteered care from families as possible. The dual roles—sometimes dubbed as advocate and gatekeeper roles—constitute a recipe for cognitive dissonance and ethical confusion (Kane, 1992a, 1992b).

People with the job title of case manager are found in many settings. In most states, a statewide program of case-managed long-term care has been created with lead agencies distributed around the state—perhaps in health departments, aging departments, human service departments, or in specially designated and contracted lead agencies, which may differ from county to county. At the same time, many hospitals, home care programs, family service agencies, mental health clinics, and even banks and financial institutions have developed case management programs for particular clientele. Also, a growing group of privately practicing case managers are becoming visible, especially in geographical areas with many retirees. Such case managers may be hired by worried out-of-town relatives to look in on their older family members and supervise their care.

Although case management is still emerging as a professional technology (Applebaum & Austin, 1990; Davies & Challis, 1986; Rose, 1992; Steinberg & Carter, 1982; Weil, Karls, & Associates, 1985), the luxury of waiting to consider the ethical ramifications is impossible; practical problems are pressing, and case managers are, therefore, forced to consider matters of ethics and matters of competent practice simultaneously.

As a field, biomedical ethics has concentrated most on relatively clearcut medical decisions, such as are made in hospitals and doctors offices. The role and responsibility of the physician as the patient's fiduciary agent has at least been well explored, even if imperfectly understood and even though it is changing with the changing shape of medical care. The role and responsibilities of case managers is much less well understood, either by case managers themselves or their clientele. Case managers are often nurses or social workers who respond to their own professional code of ethics, but they may be neither. They typically work for agencies. The services they arrange and sometimes purchase may include health services, but typically they include a broad array of socially oriented care and services. Case managers who allocate public funds are authorized to do so under various state and federal statutes. They are in a position to influence some very important decisions, but as a group of major actors, they seem to have caught ethicists by surprise.

As the cases and commentaries that form the heart of this book suggest, the ethical principles of respect for autonomy, beneficence, and justice require particular attention and interpretation for case managers. Thought must also be given to what constitutes "virtue" for a case manager in long-term care. The ever-present tension between advocacy and gatekeeping inherent in the case manager role is the backdrop for a wide range of ethical issues. These include the following:

- Dealing with risks and with clients who choose to take risks with their health and safety
- Balancing the conflicting claims of family members and clients
- Making decisions about when a client should no longer stay at home
- Protecting confidentiality and privacy appropriately while communicating appropriately with care providers, family members, and persons in the community
- Allocating scarce services fairly
- Determining how much client preferences should be allowed to drive up costs
- Treating agency vendors fairly

Variations on these themes mean that the case manager is rarely far from an ethical dilemma. In many mature case-management programs—those that have been developing their practices and policies in long-term care for a decade or more—ethical issues have, therefore, come to the forefront. Case managers are eager to examine the ethical implications of their decisions and actions in individual cases, the ethical implications of various rules and policies, and the ethical underpinnings of resource allocation formulas. This book is a step in that direction.

REFERENCES

Applebaum, R., & Austin C. (1990). *Long-term care case management*. New York: Springer.

Davies, B., & Challis, D. (1986). *Matching resources to needs in community care*. Aldershot, Hants, UK: Gower.

Kane, R. A. (1992a). Case management in long-term care: it can be ethical and efficacious. *Journal of Case Management, 1,* 76–81.

Kane, R. A. (1992b). Ethical pitfalls on the road to high-quality managed care. In S. M. Rose (Ed.), *Case management and social work practice.* New York: Longman.

Rose, S. M. (Ed). (1992). *Case management and social work practice.* New York: Longman.

Steinberg, R. M., & Carter, G. W. (1982). *Case management and the elderly: A handbook for planning and administration of programs.* Lexington, MA: D. C. Heath.

Weil, M., Karls, J. M., & Associates. (1985). *Case management in human service practice.* San Francisco: Jossey Bass.

Chapter 2

ETHICS AND CASE MANAGEMENT:
Preliminary Results of an Empirical Study

Rosalie A. Kane, Joan Dobrof Penrod, and
Helen Q. Kivnick

Case management has become the preferred approach to planning and allocating long-term care for the elderly. Somewhat optimistically, authorities expect that case management will enhance the likelihood that elderly clients receive services to allow them to be as independent as possible and to live as they prefer. But case management also is expected to serve as a force for rationalization, equity, and cost control in distribution of community long-term care services.

As statewide case-management programs have developed and matured over the last decade or so, case managers have begun to articulate the perplexing ethical issues that arise in their work. This chapter presents results from a study that was designed to describe the ethical challenges perceived by a representative sample of case managers working in publicly subsidized case-management programs in 10 states.

METHOD

We sampled 251 case managers from 10 states—California, Delaware, Georgia, Indiana, Massachusetts, Oklahoma, Oregon, Pennsylvania,

Washington, and Wisconsin. The states were selected to represent geographical and programmatic differences, but all of the selected states had statewide, publicly funded case-management programs for long-term care. In each case, the appropriate director of the case-management program agreed to participate and provided a list of local case-management programs in the state system. We then drew a random sample of five case-management agencies, stratified to include case-management programs in both urban and rural areas. Each sampled case-management program was contacted, invited to participate, and asked to provide a list of all case managers who carry current case loads. When more than five employees fit that description, five case managers were randomly selected. The aim was to interview at least 25 case managers in each state, selected from at least five programs; when sampled rural programs had fewer than five case managers, additional programs were sampled. This procedure led to a sample of somewhat more than 25 in a few states, whereas in Delaware all 18 case managers were interviews. The final sample included 251 case managers.

Trained interviewers conducted detailed telephone interviews with the selected case managers. Basic demographic data collected included age, gender, ethnicity, religion, education, income, and length of experience as a case manager. A checklist was used to determine the type and range of case-management tasks performed by the respondent. In addition, case managers' attitudes toward aging, dependency, family responsibility, public assistance, and appropriate roles for case managers was assessed using a series of 5-point Likert scales.

The heart of the interview consisted of open-ended questions about ethical issues experienced by case managers on their jobs. To eliminate fears that their own ethics were being evaluated, we explained that, for the purposes of the study, an ethical issue was any issue that the case manager had difficulty determining what was right or proper to do. Case managers were first asked to identify ethical issues experienced in their jobs. Then they were asked about ethical issues that might arise in seven categories: divergence between the clients' interests or wishes and those of family members; divergence between clients' wishes and case managers' views of clients' needs; divergence between safety concerns and other values; client confidentiality and disclosure; interprofessional or interagency disagreements; agency policies giving rise to ethical issues; and public policies giving rise to ethical issues.

With each question, the interviewer probed for examples, pressed respondents to indicate why the example illustrated an ethical issue, and asked how respondents typically reconciled or solved issues in this category. The case manager was also asked to discuss in detail the most difficult ethical issue he or she faced as a case manager-which could be one of the cases previously mentioned. Finally, we asked a set of questions about how, if at all, case managers assessed the values and preferences of their clients; what patterns, if any, they observed in the values or preferences of their clients; and how, if at all, the client's values and preferences made a difference in the conduct of the case.

We developed a coding system for responses to the open-ended questions using six completed interviews, and tested and refined the codes using an additional group of 10 interviews. We then trained five coders on the format until they achieved reliability on several questionnaires. When in doubt of how to code an item, coders were instructed to write down the response verbatim so that the authors could recode into existing or new categories. Although this study is largely descriptive, the responses were tabulated by state, gender, age, religion, and occupational tenure as a case manager.

CASE-MANAGEMENT PRACTICE DESCRIBED

Table 2.1 describes the 251 subjects. They were mostly female and white. Their average age was 40 (with a wide range). Most were Protestants (67%) or Catholics (20%), but a substantial minority said they were atheists or agnostics (13%). The 5% in the "other" category included Jews, Mormons, Muslims, Deists, and others. The most common disciplinary preparation was social work (20% with a bachelor's in social work [BSW] and 5% with a master's in social work [MSW], but the most common preparation was a nonprofessional bachelor's degree. Ten percent had a master's degree in some related field such as counseling, psychology, theology, recreation, or education. In this sample, very few were nurses. The mean salary was relatively modest. The average case load was 63, and the range in case-load size was striking. Part of the variation in case load was accounted for because of part-time employment or case managers performing other duties besides case management. We were able to calculate a ratio of the number of cases per hour worked as a case manager for about half the sample. The average number of clients per hour was 1.7, but the range went from less than 1 per hour to 6.5.

Table 2.2 shows the functions that the respondents indicated they performed as part of their case management job. More than 90% indicated that they performed certain functions that are often viewed as part of the job definition such as assessments, care planning, monitoring in persons and by phone, and reassessment, and 99% indicate that they sought to involve family members in the client's care plan. Other items

TABLE 2.1
Characteristics of 251 Case Managers and Work Conditions

Characteristic	
Gender	
Female	87%
Male	13
Average age	40 years[a]
Education	
No post–high school	6%
BSW	20
Other bachelor's degree	51
MSW	5
Other master's degree	10
Nursing degree	2
Other	6
Race[b]	
White, not Hispanic	84%
African-American	12
Native American	1
Asian/Pacific Island	1
Hispanic	2
Other	1
Religion	
Protestant	57%
Catholic	20
None	16
Other	5
No response	2
Average yearly salary[c]	$21,398
Tenure as a case manager	
2 years or less	33%
2–5 years	31
Greater than 5 years	36
Average tenure as a case manager[b]	6 years
Average current case load[e]	63 clients
Agency location	
Rural	53%
Urban	47

[a]Range = 21–68; standard deviation = 11. [b]Percentages do not add to 100 because of rounding errors. [c]Range = $11,760–40,000. [d]Range = 3 weeks to 25 years. [e]Range = 5–404 clients.

TABLE 2.2
Reported Responsibilities of Case Managers

Case manager responsibility	% ($n = 251$)
Prepare client care plan	99
Seek family participation in care plan	99
Monitor client in person	98
Refer clients who are ineligible	94
Perform comprehensive client assessments	92
Complete reassessments	91
Monitor clients by phone	91
Recommend service providers	84
Purchase services or authorize purchase for client	79
Calculate cost of services in care plan	75
Make nursing home placements	73
Determine initial eligibility	67
Develop unorthodox service arrangements when needed	64
Perform screening or intake	63
Complete case management for clients in other residential settings	63
Provide direct counseling	58
Transport or accompany client to appointment	43
Complete case management for clients in nursing home	40
Screen for nursing home preadmission	28
Provide direct personal care (e.g., nursing)	9

had less consensus, but as many as 84% recommended service providers, 79% had purchase authority; 75% calculated the cost of the care plans; and 73% made nursing home placements. About two thirds did case finding or screening, and indicated that they developed creative and unorthodox plans (e.g., finding a lawyer for a client, paying someone to walk a dog, arranging unusual home repairs). Thus, there was considerable agreement on the role of the case manager. Three functions were done by fewer than one half but more than one third of the case managers: direct counseling of clients (58%), transporting clients directly in their cars (43%), and providing case management for clients in nursing homes (40%).

Table 2.3 depicts the respondents' attitudes to a group of statements to which they could agree or disagree, and which were presented at the end of the interview. As Table 2.3 shows, respondents resoundingly endorsed the proposition that they should be advocates for getting services to clients, but about two thirds endorsed the sometimes conflicting proposition that case managers have a responsibility to see that

TABLE 2.3

Case Managers' General Attitudes

Attitude	Strongly agree (%)	Agree (%)	Neutral (%)	Disagree (%)	Strongly disagree (%)
In general, families should provide most care for their frail elderly relatives	12	37	22	23	5
Case managers should involve family members in care of elderly	79	19	1	1	
It is safer for case managers to arrange home care from an agency than from an independent vendor	36	28	21	13	2
Case managers should be advocates for getting service to clients	94	6			
If clients do not want family members involved in their care, they have a right to keep them out of it	63	30	3	2	
Case managers have responsibility to see that taxpayer's money for long-term care is wisely spent	67	20	6	5	1
If the case management program does not allow enough care to keep clients safely at home, the program should withdraw services altogether	9	12	11	26	42
If cognitively intact clients want to take risks, it is their own decision	62	27	2	5	4
If at all possible, people should have the right to die at home	87	11	1	1	

the taxpayer's money is well spent. They strongly endorsed the idea that case managers should involve family members in the care of their elderly relatives, yet they also supported the idea that family members should be able to keep their relatives out of the situation if they so prefer. Almost 50% held the general view that families *should* provide most of the care received by frail elderly persons. And, although the right to die at home received strong approval, 21% felt that if the case-management program couldn't arrange enough services for the client to be safe, it should withdraw services altogether. Responses to these questions reveal the binds inherent in case managers' jobs. Eight percent of the case managers indicated that some other specific belief guided their work. These tended to be religious beliefs in providence, or maxims such as "treating others as they would wish to be treated themselves."

ETHICAL ISSUES

Table 2.4 presents the ethical issues mentioned by the respondents in response to a first general question about the kinds of ethical problems they encounter as case managers. The classification is somewhat one of "apples and oranges," because it reflects the way respondents put the issue. Some respondents characterized ethical issues rather abstractly in terms of general principles, whereas others indicated topics that challenged them from an ethics standpoint. Only 4% (10 respondents) could think of no ethical issues in response to this unprompted question. Only 5% specifically identified client autonomy as an issue, although the 20% who highlighted the issue of determining when a nursing home placement is right and the 28% who mentioned client safety as an ethical issue must surely have been formulating the tradeoffs between client autonomy and other goals.

We inquired about whether the case managers experienced ethical issues in which the interests or wishes of clients were at variance with those of family members. As Table 2.5 shows, almost half described issues arising when a family member thought a nursing home was necessary, and the client and or case manager disagreed that such an admission would be in the client's best interest; only 6% mentioned the opposite conflict, in which the client wanted to enter a nursing home or protective setting, and the family member disagreed. Other disagreements between client and family concerned the amount or type of care desired at home (37%); typically family members were advocating for more services than the client wanted. Sometimes family members dis-

TABLE 2.4

Ethical Issues Experienced by Case Managers

Issue[a]	%
Admissions to nursing home, or board and care homes	29
Client safety	28
Confidentiality	20
Agency policies	10
Appropriateness of home care for client	9
Eligibility issues	9
Decisions about or for incompetent clients	9
Persuading client to accept other services (e.g., medical or mental health care, treatment for alcoholism)	7
Rights of family members	6
Conflicts within family, or between client and family	6
Persuasion of client to accept home care or services	6
Decisions about guardians or conservators	6
Money and property	6
Provider behavior	6
Maximizing client autonomy	5
Client right to die	5
Use of coercion or persuasion in "best interest" of client	4
None	4

Note. Other issues reported by fewer than 4% include multiple interests of parties, issues with physicians (3%); trusting the client, client fraud, racial issues, client wants too much (2%); client abuse, community (1% or fewer).
[a]Percents do not sum to 100 because participants can mention more than one issue.

agreed among themselves about the course of action for the client (7%), and sometimes the issue clearly involved money, usually the client's (7%). A few of the case managers (5%) described the issue as uncertainty about the proper roles of family members (e.g., "how much should we expect of a niece?").

Case managers tended to resolve these situations by supporting the preferences of competent clients. Only 7% reported instances in which they would actually overrule a competent client directly by siding with the family, but many would work try to get the client, the family, or both to change their view, or would look toward temporary solutions or compromises to mitigate conflict.

We asked whether ethical issues arose because of disparity between a client's wants and that client's needs. As Table 2.6 shows, almost one third described dilemmas wherein clients want to maintain a life-style that the case manager felt was inconsistent with their needs. Some of the examples included clients who lived antisocial or isolated life-styles;

TABLE 2.5
Ethical Issues Involving Conflict Between Client and Family and Their Resolutions

	%
Issue[a]	(n = 251)
Family wants nursing home, and client or case manager disagree	49
Family has different views from those of client (excluding nursing home placement)	37
Family has different views from those of case manager (excluding nursing home placement)	12
Disagreements among family about client	7
Conflicts of interest about money	7
Family does not want nursing home, and client or case manager disagree	6
Rights and responsibilities of families	5
Client wants more help than family is willing to provide	4
Family overprotects client	4
None in category	6
Resolutions[a]	(n = 237)
Case manager supports client preferences if client is competent	48
Case manager educates, counsels client and family toward change	24
Case manager urges or counsels family toward change	21
Case manager urges or counsels client toward change	14
Temporary or trial solution to mitigate conflict	11
Case manager overrules client preferences	7
No resolution	5

Note. Other issues mentioned: family wants to do more than case manager thinks is appropriate (2%).
Other resolutions mentioned: advises family on legal resources, provides services to ease family (2%); generally supports family, waits for crisis (1%).
[a]Percents do not sum to 100 because participants can mention more than one issue.

clients who took risks or lived unsafely; and clients who, in the opinion of the case manager, associated with harmful or exploitative people. Consistent with the findings presented previously, 28% pointed to clients who needed more home care than they wanted to accept, 18% to clients who "needed" more of other kinds of services than they wanted (e.g., medical care, mental health treatment, alcohol treatment), and 17% to clients who "needed," but didn't want to move to, a nursing home or residential setting. Only 11% mentioned dilemmas arising from clients who wanted more services than they "needed." Almost half the case managers who described conflicts between client "needs" and client "wants" resolved such situations by supporting the autonomy and

TABLE 2.6
Perceived Ethical Issues Because of Disparity Between Client Needs and Client Wants

	%
Issue[a]	$(n = 251)$
Client wants unsafe or unhealthy life-style	32
Client needs home care or more home care, and does not want it	28
Client needs and does not want nursing home or other placement	18
Client needs and does not want community services (e.g., medical or mental health care)	17
Client wants more services than case manager think are needed	11
Client needs but does not want to spend money but does	4
None in category	14
Resolution[a]	$(n = 216)$
Case manager supports client autonomy and preferences if client is competent	48
Case manager educates and counsels client toward change	45
Case manager overrules client autonomy and preferences	16
Case manager looks for a temporary or trial solution to mitigate conflict	13
Case manager uses family and others to persuade client	7
Referral to adult protective services	7
Legal recourse or remedy	6
No resolution	9

Note. Other issues reported: client will not cooperate (2%).
Other resolutions reported: waits for a crisis, talks with client to build trust (3%); closes the case (2%).
[a]Percents do not sum to 100 because participants can mention more than one issue.

preferences of the clients, but also almost half (and many of the same respondents who strove to support autonomy) also attempted to counsel or educate the client toward changing his or her stance. Only 16% indicated that sometimes they resolved the problem by directly overriding the client's preference, and 7% indicated that sometimes the resolution involved a referral to adult protective services.

Table 2.7 classifies the case managers' responses to a direct question about ethical issues arising because the goal of safety is at variance with other goals. Perhaps more than any other question, this one yielded responses that highlight the uncomfortable cognitive dissonance case managers can experience. Oddly, given their responses to other questions, 25% of the respondents indicated that they experienced no conflict of this type. (Perhaps this is related to the cognitive strategies people undertake to resolve cognitive dissonance.) Classifying the re-

TABLE 2.7

Perceived Ethical Issues in Which Safety was at Variance With Other Desirable Goals

	%
Issue	(n = 251)
Safety is viewed by case manager as primary goal	34
Safety and other goals and values are balanced	23
Safety is viewed by case manager as secondary to other goals	18
Could not classify/no response	25
Resolutions[a]	(n = 188)
Case manager educates and counsels both client and family toward safety, but no coercion	36
Case manager lets client decide/supports autonomy	33
No resolution	33
Case manager supports client safety (including legal action or adult protective service referral if necessary)	31
Case manager takes steps to reduce actual risks (e.g., increased monitoring, safety proofing)	30
Case manager supports client autonomy in principle, but client safety in practice	17
Case manager closes the case	4

Note. Other resolutions reported: waits for crisis (2%); depends on family willingness to accept risk (1%).
[a]Percents do not sum to 100 because participants can mention more than one issue.

sponses, we judged that about one third of the case managers held safety as the primary goal, 18% viewed safety as less important than other goals or values, and 23% tried to hold safety and other values in an uneasy balance.

Based on the case examples given and the resolutions described, we classified how case managers resolved such tension. Almost one third indicated that client safety comes first and, thus, they take all steps necessary to protect clients, whereas slightly more than one third indicated that they would let a competent client decide to take risks. Many indicated that they would attempt to persuade clients and family toward a safer situation, though they would not coerce the client, and 30% (including some who would ultimately accede to client's wishes, and some who would ultimately act forcibly to promote safety) would take steps to reduce the risks. Some respondents (17%) contradicted themselves by making a statement that client autonomy was more important than any other value and then describing their own actions to undermine that value to bring about a safe solution.

TABLE 2.8
Perceived Ethical Issues Involving Privacy and Confidentiality

	%
Issue	($n = 251$)
Concern about proper disclosure of client information to families	22
Concern about what information is appropriate to give agency providers	17
Concern about proper disclosure in absence of formal release from client	8
General concern that confidentiality will not be maintained	6
Case manager concern about too little information to agencies	4
None in this category	43
Resolution[a]	($n = 107$)
Case manager does not impart information without consent	58
Case manager uses judgment about what to disclose	56
Informed consent solves any problems	53
Case manager discloses with client permission	32
Case manager informs clients that others want information, and urges clients to share with family or others	8
No resolution	8

Note. Other issues reported: concern whether client knows how information is used (3%); concern about disclosure of family information to client, concern that information is kept from the case manager, confidentiality versus mandated referrals, disclosure of information to the public (2%).
Other resolutions: avoids learning confidential information, gains client trust, refers people who want confidential information to client; is discreet (3%); informs client of breaches (1%).
[a]Percents do not sum to 100 because participants can mention more than one issue.

As Table 2.8 shows, slightly more than half the respondents reported ethical conflicts over matters of confidentiality and disclosure. The most frequently expressed dilemma concerned what to disclose to family members (22%), followed by what to disclose to agency providers (17%). After that, there was little commonality in the way the issues were formulated. Eight percent were conflicted by needs or desires to disclose information before a formal release could be obtained, 6% were generally concerned about the impossibility of maintaining confidentiality, and 4% felt conflicted because they felt it right and proper to give more information to providers than they were supposed to do. More than 50% of those reporting conflicts about confidentiality use their judgments to some extent about what to disclose and to whom, but 58% will not impart information without permission. About one half volunteered that the informed consent process pointed the way to resolving any dilemmas.

Tables 2.9 and 2.10 describe the ethical issues that case managers perceive in their work with persons of other disciplines or in other agencies. As Table 2.9 shows, ethical conflicts cited most often involved the home care or home health agencies, or the paraprofessional home care workers (many of whom work for the agencies but some of whom are independently employed). Fourteen percent mentioned physicians

TABLE 2.9
Other Professionals With Whom Case Managers Have Ethical Conflicts

Conflict arises with	% ($n = 207$)
Home care personnel (except paraprofessionals)	38
Paraprofessional home care personnel	24
Physicians	14
Nurses	10
Mental health personnel	5
No specific other professional mentioned	28

Note. Other professionals with whom case managers have difficulty: adult protection services, hospital personnel (5%); Social/ Human Services (4%); other social workers (3%); nursing home personnel, Medicare/Social Security Administration, board and care/foster care workers (2%).

TABLE 2.10
Ethical Issues Raised for Case Managers in Dealing With Other Professionals or Agencies

Issue[a]	% ($n = 251$)
Disagreements about care plan	28
Case manager sees ethical problems in policies and practices of other agencies and providers	16
Attempt to maintain confidentiality/not give too much information	16
Process of dealing with fraudulent or illegal behavior of others including fulfillment of contracts	15
Others do not respect client preferences or autonomy	12
Client safety	7
Turf concerns	7
Other professionals and agencies will not take risks	6
Recommendation of specific providers	4
None	18

[a]Percents do not sum to 100 because participants can mention more than one issue.

specifically, and 10% mentioned nurses as sources of ethical conflict in collegial relationships. Table 2.10 shows little consensus among case managers about the content of ethical issues arising with other professions. Indeed, some of the issues entailed interprofessional and interagency disagreements that could readily be construed as technical practice issues in care planning. The examples offered suggest that they became ethical issues for the case manager when care providers and other agencies involved in the case face the identical ethical issues as the case manager (for instance, safety versus autonomy, or the interests of family versus the interests of clients) but resolve them differently. Then, case managers must consider whether their judgments outweigh those of other professionals. In some instances, the case managers perceived that the behavior of other agencies or personnel was not ethical. For example, a worker might be billing extra hours or a physician might have a conflict of interest in recommending a particular nursing home. The dilemma arose, in part, in determining what to do about whistle blowing.

Case managers tended to resolve these conflicting situations by efforts to negotiate and compromise (31%) and to win the confidence of their collaborators (6%). Only 10% mentioned simply overriding other providers and colleagues, though another 10% mentioned that they sometimes appealed to a higher authority or went over the head of the person causing difficulty. Although often feasible, sometimes case managers helped the client find another provider (e.g., another physician, nursing home, or home care provider) or refused to refer to that professional or organization anymore. The case descriptions showed, however, that case managers often felt it was not feasible for them to police the marketplace by blackballing providers.

Table 2.11 describes the case managers' responses to the question of whether any agency policy poses ethical questions for them as case managers, and Table 2.12 shows their responses to the question of whether any public policy poses ethical issues for them as case managers. Fewer case managers reported problems in these areas, with more than 40% indicating no problems of that sort. For example, 45% saw no agency policies that raised ethical issues, and 6% of these volunteered that theirs was a wonderful agency. There was some lack of clarity about which policies were agency policies and which were public policies. Arbitrary rules that harm clients, excessive paperwork that interferes with more important goals and values, lack of resources that lead to inadequate or inequitable service, and constraints on the case manager's professional discretion were variously interpreted as public policies, agency policies, or both. Some of this ambiguity is inevitable because case-management programs are the creature of public policy but are

TABLE 2.11
Perceived Ethical Issues Regarding Agency Policies

Issue[a]	% ($n = 251$)
None	45
Fraudulent policies	8
Eligibility for services	7
Case manager praises agency policies—no ethical issues raised	6
Excess bureaucracy	6
Excess paperwork	5
Information disclosure	4

Note. Other issues mentioned: supervisors are unethical (3%); rules for case closure, restrictions on what case managers can pay for, restrictions on what care attendants can do, underfunding (2%); restrictions on referrals, insufficient authority, case manager remuneration (1%).
[a]Percents do not sum to 100 because participants can mention more than one issue.

TABLE 2.12
Perceived Ethical Issues Regarding Public Policies

Issue[a]	% ($n = 251$)
None	41
Understaffed/underfunded programs	17
Eligibility for services	12
Excess paperwork	7
Policies compromise case manager expertise	6
Rules about covered services	6
Medicaid policies	4
Availability of home care	4
Abuse and neglect reporting and referral requirements	4

Note. Others mentioned: guardianship (3%); waiting lists, Medicare policies, inappropriate standards for case managers (2%); housing, reimbursement rates for nursing homes, expectations and rules regarding families, Title XX social services (1%).
[a]Percents do not sum to 100 because participants can mention more than one issue.

implemented through a particular agency. Also respondents may have been uncertain whether to consider that their agency included the state-level lead agency running the case-management program as internal to the agency or as makers of public policies.

We were eager to learn how case managers went about assessing the values and preferences of their clients. As Table 2.13 shows, the com-

TABLE 2.13
Approach to Assessing Clients' Values and Preferences

Approach used by case manager[a]	% (*n* = 251)
Try to get to know the client as a person	51
Ask about client's history and past	30
Ask about preferences regarding family members	25
Ask about spirituality and religion	23
Ask opinions about or reactions to proposed, actual, or past services	18
Notice things, unobtrusive observations as part of general assessment	17
Administer a series of structured questions (usually about advance directives)	16
Ask about hobbies, interests, tastes, activities	15
Ask the client's feelings about things	13
Get information from family	10
No response	2

Note. Other approaches mentioned: ask about biases (4%); ask about death, ask about money, ask about cultural background (3%); not case managers' role to assess values, life goals (2%); ask about placement satisfaction (1%).
[a]Percents do not sum to 100 because participants can mention more than one issue.

mon answers here were extremely general, one half indicated that they try to get to know the client as a person. Other general responses included asking about the client's history and past (30%), asking their feelings about things (13%), and just noticing things (17%). (Elaborations of what would be noticed included the furniture, the food, the cleanliness, and the way people behaved toward each other.) Some ask specifically for opinions about services they had received in the past or that were being contemplated for the present. Very few indicated that they would ask about preferences related to health care.

Table 2.14 reports the kinds of preferences case managers believed their clients hold. Most frequently the case managers discern that their clients prefer to remain at home and that they prefer independence. The lower part of Table 2.14 shows that 51% of case managers suggest one pattern of preference only and tend to generalize about their clients. Another 8% indicated that clients are different from each other, but specified only one set of observations. About one third mentioned more than one pattern that they had observed, for example, that some clients strongly prefer not to give trouble, whereas others like as much help as possible. Some of those went on to attribute the differences to specific factors such as ethnicity, religion, education, rural versus urban location, or personality factors. Table 2.15 shows how client preferences were believed to influence the care plans. Again the answers tended to

TABLE 2.14
Case Managers' Perceptions of Client Preferences

	%
Client preference noted by case manager[a]	($n = 251$)
Remain at home	35
Maintain independence/self-reliance	32
Have things done for him or her	14
Reject formal community services	10
Controls own life	9
Exist without welfare or government help	6
Maintain privacy	6
Have own money/enough money and possessions	6
Have family help	5
No response	12
Variations reported by case managers	
Single pattern of preferences applying to all clients	51
Different preferences presented	31
Different preferences but no specifics presented	8
No response	10

Note. Other issues: prefer not to be involved with strangers, prefer family help, protect family/not have help from family, concerned about money and possessions, have minimal help (5%); maintain dignity (3%); prefer being useful/having a purpose in life to having government help, continuity with life-style/no changes (2%).
[a]Percentages do not sum to 100 because participants can mention more than one item.

TABLE 2.15
Influence of Client Preferences on Care Plans

	%
Influence[a]	($n = 251$)
Type of care/help arranged	48
Nothing specific is mentioned, but case manager reports preferences do influence	21
Client preference does not influence care plan	16
Scheduling of help or care	12
Case manager will change plan if client is dissatisfied	8
Racial and ethnic concerns and needs	6
Respect preferences for race of formal helper	4
No response	4

Note. Other influences: placement in nursing home or other residence, choice of particular nursing home (2%); choice of guardian (1%).
[a]Percents do not sum to 100 because participants can mention more than one issue.

be vague; 16% said client preferences had little effect, 21% merely said they influenced the care plan but could offer no details when probed, and 48% said they influenced the broad types of care arranged (e.g., home care versus day care, community-based care versus nursing home care). Eight percent indicated that if the client expressed a preference against the plan *after* it is put in place, they will make a change.

Table 2.16 shows what processes or approaches the case managers take generally to resolve ethical issues. The table reveals that there are few institutionalized or systematic processes to assist case managers. Most resolve it themselves or do so in discussion with supervisors or colleagues, or both. A few have consultants or training available or resort to the agency's legal counsel.

We also coded the entire interview for the presence or absence of particular themes of interest to us, such as racial issues, issues involving physicians, or issues involving community pressures on the case manager. About half the interviews (49%) contained issues of conflict between clients and family members. About a quarter described one or more ethical issues arising from conflict with the policies of their own agency (27%) or because of issues involving racial or ethnic differences (26%). Twenty percent of those interviewed cited an ethical issue arising from their work with physicians, and 12% cited one or more issues in which the case manager was caught between client interests and community standards.

Case Examples

The case examples provided by the respondents to illustrate each category of dilemma and as their most difficult ethical problem were vividly described. They were also complex and difficult to resolve. The cases for which we have solicited commentaries (and which are found in Part II of this book) are drawn directly from the responses with slight changes for the purpose of anonymity.

CONCLUSION

Our findings suggest that, as we had suspected, case management is indeed an ethical mine field. The respondents were generally conscious of struggling with difficult decisions involving important choices in their client's lives. In some instances, we as researchers perceived an ethical conflict where the case manager perceived none, or we framed the

TABLE 2.16
Case Managers' Approaches to Resolving Ethical Dilemmas

Approach[a]	% ($n = 251$)
Discussion with supervisors	68
Discussion with colleagues	39
Case and care conference	17
Resolution alone	10
No response	8
Inservice training	4
Legal counsel	4

Note. Other resolutions mentioned: use of outside consultants, help from administrator, consult higher administrative level in state (3%); consult manual rules, ethics committee (2%); mandated reports, consult board of directors (1%).
[a]Percents do not sum to 100 because participants can mention more than one issue.

ethical problems differently from the way the case manager did. Regardless of the ethics spin put on the problem, however, one is impressed after reading these interviews that case managers consciously experience ethical dilemmas. Many case managers are losing sleep worrying about whether they are doing the right thing for and about their clients.

One case manager summarized it poignantly by a comment that she was expected to be all things to all people—to serve clients, family members, provider agencies, and the general community—and that doing it right was difficult. Case managers were particularly conflicted about what to do in cases of marginal competency (which apparently abound) and in how to define competence in the first place. Although fewer case managers presented organizational and policy themes, taken as a whole substantial numbers of respondents were concerned that their eligibility policies or their service limits were somehow unfair. Some felt that the whole program was a "false promise" because of its underfunding. Substantial numbers felt they had insufficient professional discretion to make decisions, yet they freely acknowledged that even with discretion, they often did not know what they should do.

The difficulty for case managers is exacerbated because they have the constant sense of dealing with important life-and-death matters in an imperfect world.

146,184

PART II

CASES AND COMMENTARIES

Chapter 3

ABOUT THE CASES

Rosalie A. Kane and Arthur L. Caplan

The cases presented here all originated from the interview study described in chapter 2. We fictionalized the details, but the themes are recognizable. From the many poignant and challenging cases presented to us, we chose those that represent frequently occurring types of problems, but we also endeavored to present the range of issues. More than one client and family situation tends to be depicted within a single "case."

At least two (and in two instances three) commentaries are provided for each case. This luxury affords a view of how different ethicists with different disciplinary backgrounds and theoretical bents construe the issues in a particular case. We were particularly eager to show multiple perspectives because the area of case management is so new to ethics exploration. Brief reactions from persons administering case-management programs at the state (and in one case, local) level are also included.

Arranging the cases was somewhat challenging because no particular logical order stands out as best, though we tried to move from the particular to the more general. The first two cases deal with risks of one sort or another. Deciding what risks clients should be permitted to take, whether case managers have the responsibility to protect their clients from risks, or, conversely, whether they have no right to do so is the ordinary stuff of a case manager's day. In chapter 4, Brian Hofland and Carol Tauer deal with the kinds of risky cases that case managers confront, often with a need to make a quick decision with insufficient information about the risks themselves, or even about the competence of the client to understand the risks. Hofland suggests an orderly approach to discerning the relevant facts and weighing risks in the service of promoting autonomy, and Tauer further distinguishes between risks and choices in the situations of the three clients. Synthesizing the views of administrators and case managers in the huge California system of case-managed care, Patrick Murphy endorses a modest and realistic view of the role and power of the case manager, all of which would be used to support client choice as much as possible.

In the next grouping in chapter 5, Susan Wolf and Muriel Ryden, an attorney and nurse, respectively, each comment on a case involving one client who is marginally competent and one who is *clearly* incompetent but whose family judges that the risks of being locked at home alone are preferable to placement in a nursing home. Wolf uses this vehicle to explore whether case managers have a fiduciary duty to their clients, similar to the trust relationship between physicians and clients. She concludes they do—but that they must act within a system with safeguards. Ryden examines the same cases and develops a line of moral reasoning that might assist case managers in making fine distinctions. In these instances, the two reactors, both nurses who administer large case-management programs in Minneapolis and Oklahoma, respectively, would not countenance a case manager's decision to leave a demented woman in a locked home for hours at a time. Monson suggests some practical tests of true risk (Can she dial 911 for help? Does she open the door to strangers?). He also suggests that plans could be made that are much less restrictive or alien than admission to a nursing home yet still protective.

Chapter 6 contains commentaries from three philosophers on a prototypical case of eccentric clients, those whose life-styles may offend the community and even the case manager. Baruch Brody argues that the public does indeed have an interest in some degree of conformity to conventions. He also asserts the concept that competence, so often unclear in these situations, must be judged on a decision-by-decision basis. Dr. Brody introduces a possible virtue in case managers-that is, being imaginative. Bart Collopy's commentary tackles the cases of these eccentrics through an exploration of beneficence. Collopy contends that this principle precludes abandoning clients even if they reject most of the care we offer. He derives a moral requirement for the watchful waiting strategies used by so many of the case managers we surveyed.

Stephen Post explores the tensions between the person and the community that may arise as older people cling to particular places that offer a sense of continuity with their pasts. This case resonates with case managers, almost all of whom have one or more "cat ladies" among their clientele. They typically also have one or more clients who have lived on the fringes of society all their lives—perhaps as hermits, perhaps as part of a counterculture—and are uncertain how to approach "standards" for their care.

Chapter 7, "Fault Lines," takes the question of risk a step further, and introduces the possibility that family members are being exploitative, neglectful, or abusive. As Adrienne Asch and Rebecca Dresser comment on this case, the complexities of labeling a family as neglectful or exploitative become apparent. Things are rarely that clearcut. At the same time Asch raises a provocative question about the assumptions about a family that undergird long-term care programs. She suggests that the help and assistance needed by people with disabilities is better provided by persons other than relatives so that true distinctions can be maintained between reciprocal relationships of caring and affecting, and "care" in the sense of instrumental help. Both Asch and Dresser, an attorney, use these cases to point to systemic problems in guardianship and protective programs. It is intriguing that they both begin their commentaries with a reminiscence of their own earlier experiences as social workers, and express admiration for those who can withstand the difficulties and ambiguities of the case-manager role. Despite this empathy, however, both these commentaries rail against the assumptions that disability equals incompetence and that older people cannot speak for themselves. Dresser also suggests that there are subtle and not-so-subtle issues of sexism in the way the problems presented in this case were formulated and handled. Finally, she raises the concern that, if professionals fail to understand their own values, they may act to meet their personal needs rather than those of the clients.

Looming on the horizon for all community long-term care clients is the prospect that they might someday be destined to enter a nursing home. When home care becomes too expensive or too risky, a nursing home may be recommended. In chapter 8, Arthur Caplan and Rebecca Elon comment on this emotionally laden topic; in different ways, each approaches the question of whether a nursing home admission need always be a bad outcome. Caplan's essay attacks as a delusion the notion that case managers can ever be acting in a client's best interest by consigning him or her to a nursing home as we know it today. Elon broadens the discussion to consider "death" as an outcome of all our endeavors. She proposed that the hospice philosophy (even if death is not immediately imminent) might be a useful perspective for case managers, given its emphasis on maintaining meaning in life rather than postponing death and disability. Finally, just as Asch questioned the term "care" in the previous chapter, here Elon questions the term "placement," with its imagery of storing inanimate objects, and suggests that cleaning up our language could lead to more sensitivity in practice.

Confidentiality and disclosure—when to tell, whom to tell, when not to tell, whom not to tell—constitute perennial issues for case managers, who must deal with collecting and exchanging information in a routine way. In chapter 9, Amitai Etzioni and Rosalie Kane explore ethical issues involved in exchanging or withholding information. Etzioni argues that a caring community, as opposed to governments, often has a stake in knowing about its members, and that privacy is not the most critical principle. Kane, in contrast, suggests that autonomy (as well as trust) is often best served by keeping confidence, and presents a nuanced approach to considering what to tell and why.

Chapter 10 brings us into an arena in which the work of the individual case manager is molded by organizational context. Case-management programs that allocate benefits typically function within rules that can readily seem arbitrary and capricious. Mary Mahowald uses civil disobedience analogies to explore the ethics of breaking the rules in individual cases while respecting the rules, a paradox also taken up in Kathleen Powderly's comment on the same case.

Case managers attain power in their communities. They send business in the direction of various agencies and care providers. They pay for services and expect accountability for quality and price. Conversely, providers have their own professional ethics and professional self-interests to protect (and sometimes the former and the latter can get somewhat muddled). In chapter 11, Don Postema and Joan Penrod explore the ethics of the relationship between case managers and providers. In the name of ethics, Postema calls for collegiality, which in turn modifies the stance of case managers who would call all the shots. Penrod analyzes the multiple dilemmas from the standpoint of skilled practice, within a framework of respect for the autonomy of competent adults. Both suggest that tact, diplomacy, human relations skill, and communication might go a way to averting ethical dilemmas.

Chapter 12 takes us into a touchy and painful issue—the extent to which the preferences of a client should be honored when preference is barely indistinguishable from prejudice. Clients may insist on white caregivers, for example. Three commentaries are offered—Reinhard Priester provides a legal perspective, and Oliver Williams offers a social work perspective; their conclusions differ somewhat. Priester refers to evolving law on discrimination in employment, and Williams calls for "ethically proficient" case managers, who can learn to distinguish between culturally relevant preferences and unjustified prejudice. His arguments would lead to greater deference to the preference of an Afro-American for a worker of her own race than the preference of a white for a white worker. Adrienne Asch draws on her perspective as a civil rights activist in a provocatively titled commentary: "Free to Be a Bigot." She argues that the very nature of the relationship between a disabled person, and his or her assistant requires that idiosyncratic client preferences on a range of matters, including race and gender of the assistant, be honored as much as practically feasible.

Finally, chapter 13 introduces a plethora of "macroissues," all related to fairness in the allocation of services. Who gets what, who gets served from the waiting list first—these are the concerns not only of the line case manager, but also of those who design and operate the system. Miles promulgates some general guidelines, and Post focuses particularly on fairness regarding expectations held for family members to be part of the caring system.

Taken cumulatively, these 10 cases illustrate the breadth and depth of the difficult ethical issues in case management and community long-term care. They also put some flesh on ethical abstractions. The problems presented here occur in families, in communities, and in work groups, as the vivid words of clients and case managers remind us. Each chapter concludes with some questions for further discussion, which were provided by the editors. Undoubtedly both ethicists and case managers will be able to elaborate on both the questions and the answers.

Chapter 4

RISKY BUSINESS: Who Decides on What Risks?

CASE

■

Mrs. D lives in a two-bedroom apartment. She needs complete help with transferring out of bed, bathing, and other personal care. She is receiving this help from a middle-aged woman who has been well known to her over the years and is sort of a friend. Mrs. D's daughter wants her to come and live with her in another part of the state, but Mrs. D wants to stay where she is.

Mrs. D's caregiver gives meticulous care, and the client is always clean and turned. No infections or bedsores have occurred despite the fact that Mrs. D is at risk for such problems. But the caregiver has two sons, both of whom have had brushes with the law. One is reputed to be using cocaine. Both sons have moved in with their mother and Mrs. D. The case manager also thinks that this caregiving family is exploiting Mrs. D financially when they cash her checks and buy her groceries. Mrs. D refuses to press charges. It is her money and her life, and she says this is the best situation for her. She seems competent, but who knows? Would a normal person want to live this way? What is the case manager's responsibility to the client? To the daughter who calls frequently? Mrs. D has enjoined the case manager not to discuss the details with her daughter, and so far the case manager has acquiesced.

If the case manager wanted to she could finesse this ethical problem. After all, cocaine use is illegal. But the case is so similar to so many others.

The case manager also has Mr. K to think about. He has no nearby relatives, and he needs so much more care than the program can offer. He lives out in the country with a wood-burning stove, and he won't be able to bring in the wood next winter in his present condition. Various neighbors help, but they can't really be responsible. Recently he fell and was on the floor for 19 hours before a neighbor found him. He was hospitalized with a fractured hip, but he insisted on leaving the facility and going back home as soon as he could hobble. The case manager is strongly considering telling the neighbors not to help him to bring it to a head but so far has not.

They also need to think of Miss J. There is no inadequacy in Miss J's living or care situation. She cooperates completely with the care plan, and her home is comfortable and clean. Miss J has a deteriorating illness and has told the case manager that she plans to end her life when she decides the time has come, and certainly "long before anyone suggests a nursing home." Miss J says, "I have a gun and I know how to use it."

COMMENTARIES

Use of Facts to Resolve Conflicts Between Beneficence and Autonomy

■

Brian F. Hofland

BACKGROUND

These three case vignettes provide classic examples of clashes between the ethical principles of beneficence and autonomy. In each vignette, there exists a conflict between the client's understanding of what is in her or his best interest, and the case manager's understanding of what is in the best interest of the client. Unfortunately, in home care the perspective of the case manager is often the only one considered. The personal autonomy of the older client frequently is seriously and unduly constricted with options that are severely restricted and inappropriate, and with a paternalistic agency deciding the particulars of care.

Kane and her colleagues (1990) pointed out that, from an ethical perspective, it is clear that long-term care for older clients should be arranged in ways that are much more respectful of their personal autonomy There are necessary limits to that autonomy. Impaired capacity for decision making can limit the individual's potential for autonomy, and many older adults in long-term care do need protection. Also, respect for autonomy is no panacea. Autonomous living inevitably entails negotiation, compromise, and accommodation. Autonomy is an important and often overlooked value in long-term care, but it is not a supreme value that trumps all others.

Yet, how we view and value aging and the aged centrally influences the goals that we set for or allow older adults, and the extent to which autonomy is supported in case-management practice. Our treatment of older adults differs from our treatment of younger adults in our willingness, with elders, to abandon autonomy in the name of protection. If the three case examples provided were changed to involve situations with younger publicly supported clients with physical disabilities, would the question of need for paternalistic intervention from the case worker even arise? Probably not. In an ageist fashion, there is a willingness to take away or restrict the freedoms and autonomy of older home care clients supposedly to "protect" them.

Even for the case manager committed to the enhancement of client autonomy, the complexity of the very concept of autonomy makes the task of coordinating care in an autonomy-enhancing manner a very delicate and difficult one. Collopy (1990) made a useful distinction between negative and positive autonomy. A negative definition of autonomy prohibits case managers from interfering with the decisions or behavior of the elderly. A positive definition of autonomy would require case mangers to provide resources and assistance, and to advocate for the elderly in an effort to enlarge and enhance their autonomy. A purely negative view of autonomy can result in a kind of cruel abandonment of the elderly to their own choices and behavior. As Kapp (1989) commented:

> [P]ower over one's life entails more than mere control over particulars of choice. In a real sense, it is knowledge that creates power. Hence, the older individual's purported right to make choices about matters affecting him or her acquires meaning only if those choices are accompanied by adequate information, both about the personal rights involved and the factual ramifications of one's decision, as well as the range of reasonable alternatives among which to choose. (p. 5)

Thus, positive autonomy requires not only that case managers allow autonomous choice, but that they actively enhance it and find ways for it to flourish among the elderly.

An understanding of positive autonomy is certainly relevant to these three case vignettes and moderates somewhat the classic adversarial clash between the ethical principles of beneficence and autonomy. In the name of autonomy, there are instances in which active involvement and even intervention in client choices are appropriate.

Necessary limits to autonomy include the competition of the interests of one client with those of other clients and caregivers, impaired capacity for decision making, and the valid need of some clients for protection. However, even when a decidedly paternalistic stance by the case manager is legitimized by the need to remove the older adult from clear and immediate danger or reduce the risk to such danger, the case-management strategy should be guided by "the principle of maximizing risk reduction using the least restrictive and least intensive care plan options" (Hennessy, 1989, p. 636).

CASE ANALYSES

In an ethical analysis of any case, there are at least four useful steps. First, what are the facts about the case (or to use a term of ethicists, the "is")? Second, what ethical principles are involved in the case? Third, are any of the facts in the case amenable to change so that the application of the ethical principles is clarified and simplified? Fourth, given the application of these principles what should the practitioner, or in these instances the case manager, do (what is the "ought")?

The Case of Mr. K

Let's take the easiest case first, that of Mr. K. What are the facts?

1. Mr. K has no nearby relatives.
2. He needs more care than the service program can offer.
3. He lives in the country.
4. He has only a wood-burning stove.
5. He won't be able to bring in the wood for his stove next winter.
6. Various neighbors help Mr. K, but can't be expected to be responsible for round-the-clock supervision.
7. A recent fall resulted in a fractured hip and the fall was undiscovered for 19 hours.
8. Mr. K has a strongly stated preference for remaining in his home despite the risk of falls.
9. There is no evidence of decisional incapacity on the part of Mr. K.

The ethical principles involved in the case are a fairly clearcut conflict between beneficence and autonomy, between the best interests definition of the case manager for Mr. K and the best interests definition of Mr. K for himself. Because there is no evidence of decisional incapacity, the case manager has an obligation to uphold the stated preference of Mr. K if at all possible. Of course, the case manager should first make sure that the strong preference of Mr. K is based on thorough awareness and knowledge of the alternative living arrangements and options that may be available to him. If not, she has an obligation to provide him with this information. Let's assume that Mr. K has this information. Rather than abandon him to his choices, however, the case manager should invoke a positive sense of autonomy, provide resources and assistance, and advocate for him so that his choice of remaining in his rural home is one that allows him to flourish.

Under no circumstances should the case manager tell the neighbors not to help Mr. K so that a crisis is precipitated and the case manager's definition of Mr. K's best interests implemented and enforced. This heavy-handed approach would violate the basic ethical principle of nonmaleficence; the case manager should do no harm to her client. Clients have quite enough crises in their lives without case managers introducing additional ones to prove a point.

Which facts are most amenable to change so that this ethical parsing can be applied? Two facts particularly appear malleable. The fact that Mr. K has only a wood-burning stove that would require endless, physically taxing several-times-daily wood-carrying trips presents a major barrier to the enhancement of Mr. K's autonomy yet is relatively easily surmountable. Does Mr. K have any assets that could be used to purchase an oil-burning stove so that he does not have to bring in wood and increase his risk of falling? Would his relatives who live some distance away be willing to purchase and install an oil-burning stove? Does the service program have the flexibility to purchase a new stove, or are there other entitlement programs or resources that could be marshaled to purchase the stove? Could the case manager interest a local service club such as Rotary, Lion's, Kiwanis, or Mr. K's church, or any nearby church to take on the purchase of the stove as a worthwhile project? Perhaps a local merchant or supplier would be willing to sell the stove at cost. The case manager is limited in invoking a positive sense of autonomy and advocating for the client only by the extent of her creativity, time, and energy.

The second fact that can easily be changed is that a fall need not go undiscovered for 19 hours. The purchase and installation of one of the relatively inexpensive, but high-quality and flexible, medical alert systems now available could allow Mr. K to signal if and when he has a fall so that he could receive prompt attention. If it is not possible or practical for a hospital or service agency to serve as the monitor for the system, perhaps a neighbor or neighbors would be willing to have the system keyed into their homes so that they could provide timely assistance. The willingness of neighbors to help Mr. K is a valuable resource that should be encouraged in creative ways by the case manager to maximize Mr. K's autonomy rather than be discouraged. The financing of the medical alert system could be pursued through the same kind of options as indicated for the oil-burning stove. Perhaps a formal medical alert system is not necessary, and the same effect could be achieved by mobilizing relatives and neighbors to telephone Mr. K once or twice a day. If he does not answer the call, a personal visit to check out his situation could be made.

By modifying these facts through active involvement and even mild intervention by the case manager, Mr. K's preference of remaining in the home can be upheld with a reduction in his risk for falls. Risk reduction has been achieved by using the least restrictive and least intensive care plan options. The case is the simplest from an ethical sense because client risk is primarily a function of service program resource limitations rather than client choices that are fraught with the potential for self-harm. Reduction of risk in the case of Mr. K is primarily a logistical exercise in overcoming resource barriers rather than an issue of overriding client choice and autonomy. What is needed most from the case manager is a great deal of creativity and ingenuity.

Case of Mrs. D

One of the key issues in the case of Mrs. D is that not all of the critical facts have been ascertained or clarified. The case manager is reacting at least partially to rumor and innuendo.

Among the facts that have been established are the following:

1. Mrs. D lives in a two-bedroom apartment.
2. She needs complete help with transferring out of bed, bathing, and other personal care.
3. She receives excellent, meticulous care from a middle-aged woman who she's known for years and is sort of a friend.
4. The caregiver has two sons who have moved in with Mrs. D and their mother.
5. The case manager thinks that the caregiving family is financially abusing Mrs. D, but Mrs. D refuses to press charges, stating that the caregiving situation is the best one for her.

6. Mrs. D's daughter wants Mrs. D to come and live with her in another part of the state.
7. Mrs. D wants to stay where she is rather than live with her daughter.
8. Mrs. D has asked the case manger not to discuss details of her situation with her daughter; to date the case manager has not.

Information that needs to be better established or clarified includes what is meant by the two sons' "brushes with the law." Does this refer to misdemeanors such as minor traffic violations, or to felonies such as income tax evasion, forcible rape, ax murders, or to what? Have the two sons been accused of crimes or actually convicted? The answers to these questions make a big difference in how this case is analyzed. Similarly, one son "is reputed to be using cocaine." Who has made this accusation? What evidence is there to support it? Has the case manager actually asked Mrs. D if this is true? Unless this rumor can be substantiated as a fact, the case manger should not include it as a factor in her case analysis. The case manager "thinks" that the caregiver family is financially exploiting Mrs. D. Does she have any evidence to support this hypothesis, or is it simply based on her dislike for the caregiver's two sons? If Mrs. D thinks that she is not being exploited and is receiving good "care value" for the money that she is spending on the caregiver family, can exploitation actually be occurring? It seems at least partly to be a matter of interpretation.

The ethical principles involved in this case again center on a conflict between beneficence and autonomy. Although there is no evidence for decisional incapacity on the part of Mrs. D, the case manager has called her competency into question, primarily because Mrs. D's choices and life-style are different from those that the case manager would opt for and because Mrs. D has refused interventions recommended by the case manager. A fact that should be added to this case is the lack of evidence of decisional incapacity on the part of Mrs. D.

A more pertinent question than whether Mrs. D's autonomy is competent or incompetent is whether her autonomy is authentic or inauthentic (Collopy, 1990). Does her stated preference to remain in her present caregiving situation reflect her identity, personal history, and values? Or is it the result of coercion that she feels because of a perception that her only alternatives are to live with a daughter that she perhaps does not like in a strange city that she does not know or to live in a nursing home in her own city? Does she have thorough awareness and knowledge of other alternative living arrangements and options that are available to her? Did she state her preference to the case manager in private, or was she fearful of possible retaliation from an eavesdropping caregiver family? If Mrs. D's decision is competent and authentic, then the case manager is faced with an exceedingly grave burden of justification for any intervention against that decision (Collopy, 1988).

A final ethical issue in this case is: Who is the client? The case manager may feel some pressure from the frequent calls and questions by Mrs. D's daughter. Clearly Mrs. D is the client, and the case manager's primary responsibility is to her. Mrs. D has asked the case manager not to discuss details of the caregiving situation with the daughter, and the case manager appropriately has not done so. She should continue not to do so and should recommend that the daughter talk directly to her mother.

Three facts are perhaps amenable to change in this case. First, the caregiver has two sons who have moved in with Mrs. D and their mother. If the sons have been convicted of serious, violent crimes and if one son is a crack addict (however, these facts would have to be established), then Mrs. D is in clear and immediate danger. The case manger would be justified in overriding Mrs. D's preference and insisting that either the two sons move out or public funds for this particular caregiver will be cut off. Second, if the caregiver family is financially exploiting Mrs. D, the case manager might be able to negotiate an agreement with Mrs. D in which a representative payee would be named to handle her financial affairs. In this way, the two functions of personal care and financial management would be disaggregated and handled by different caregiver parties. The opportunity for financial exploitation would end. Finally, the daughter's concerns about her mother are understandable. The case manager could obtain permission from Mrs. D to relate to the daughter the excellent personal care that her mother is receiving from the caregiver. Also, the case manager could try to arrange a joint meeting between Mrs. D, her daughter, and the case manager to discuss concerns.

Once many of the facts in this case have been clarified, the specific course of action that should be pursued by the case manager will also become clearer. If Mrs. D's decision to remain in her present caregiving situation is competent and authentic, however, the burden of justification for any intervention by the case manager is substantial.

Case of Miss J

The facts in this case are rather sparse.

1. There is no inadequacy in Miss J's living or care situation, her home is comfortable and clean.

2. She cooperates completely with the care plan.
3. She has a deteriorating illness.
4. She has told the case manager that she plans to end her life when she decides the time has come.
5. She states that she has a gun and knows how to use it.

Several facts need to be clarified in the case. What is the nature of the deteriorating illness of Miss J? Does she have Alzheimer's disease or a related dementia? Does she fear the loss of her mental capacity or institutionalization? These fears could be allayed perhaps by knowledge about and implementation of advance directives and reassurance about and a visit to a nursing home that provides excellent care and will accept Miss J as a resident when the time comes. Does she have a disease that causes her severe pain that she fears will worsen? This fear could be removed through proper knowledge and implementation of good pain management. Is Miss J depressed? Depression can be treated through psychological and pharmacological therapies. Finally, does Miss J actually have a gun? This fact needs to be established at once. If Miss J has Alzheimer's disease, she is not only at high risk of killing herself, but also of injuring caregivers and family members (Lecso, 1989).

The ethical principles involved are a conflict between beneficence and autonomy. Because there is a clear and immediate danger to Miss J's life, the case manager is justified in overriding Miss J's autonomy to protect her. A relevant distinction in this case is that between immediate and long-range autonomy (Collopy, 1990). If Miss J's immediate autonomy is upheld and she kills herself, she has eliminated any possibility for long-range autonomy. The case manager, by intervening, will actually be more respectful of Miss J's autonomy in the long-term sense. Two facts are amenable to change. First, Miss J may no longer want to end her life if the case manger provides Miss J with knowledge about and implementation of treatment and intervention options such as advance directives, pain management, therapy for depression, and hospice care. Second, if Miss J has Alzheimer's disease or a related dementia and does indeed have a gun, she will no longer have if it is removed from her home.

The case manger should take immediate and strong action in this case. Suicide threats should never be taken lightly or ignored. The chances are high that Miss J's threat is a desperate cry for help and does not represent an authentic desire to end her life. If she truly wanted to commit suicide, she would keep the idea to herself and just do it. The fact that Miss J has shared this information with the case manager radically changes their relationship. The case manager has a responsibility to use her creativity to uncover the issues and fears that are causing

Miss J to make her extreme threat. If necessary and available, community mental health professionals need to be involved. At the same time, the fact that a suicide threat has been made puts Miss J at considerable risk of a suicide attempt or actual suicide, as mental health experts will attest. Miss J is in great danger.

Others may argue that suicide is a rational, authentic, and reasonable decision for Miss J, but it is beyond the scope of this commentary to articulate and discuss this position fully. Beyond the moral repugnancy with which many view suicide, however, the great danger in advocating the right to suicide is that in an ageist society that devalues older people with disabilities, the right to die can become a duty to die. As geriatrician Joanne Lynn (personal communication, 1989) has noted, the desire for assisted suicide among some older people is a stinging indictment of our health care system. Individuals would rather die than have to go through the inhumane care that is provided. Advocacy by professionals of the "right" to suicide for older adults can be in truth a cynical abandonment of the older client and an abdication of professional responsibility to improve our systems of care.

In the case of Miss J, suffice it to say that the case manager has an ethical responsibility to see to it that her client does not kill herself or others. She needs to discover what is prompting this suicide threat, educate Miss J about alternative resources and care plan options, involve other professionals when appropriate, and, if Miss J is suffering from dementia, remove any gun from her home.

CONCLUSION

Autonomy can be a source of continuing and important ethical conflict between older home care clients and the case managers who coordinate their care. To the extent that case management tries to protect clients from their own foolish or harmful choices, this protection comes at high cost of client individuality and freedom. In the face of clear and immediate danger to the client, autonomy may seem like a superfluous benefit. Particularly in instances in which a client decision is both competent and authentic, a heavy burden of justification for interventions against and compromises in client autonomy lies with the case manager. When such actions are indeed justified, the guiding principle should be the maximization of risk reduction using the least restrictive and least intensive care options possible. Also, a positive sense of autonomy requires that case managers not only allow autonomous client choice, but that they actively work to enhance client autonomy and allow it to flourish.

REFERENCES

Collopy, B. J. (1988). Autonomy in long term care: Some crucial distinctions. *The Gerontologist, 28* (Suppl.), 10–17.

Collopy, B. J. (1990). Ethical dimensions of autonomy in long term care. *Generations, 14* (Suppl.), 9–12.

Hennessy, C. H. (1989). Autonomy and risk: The role of client wishes in community-based long-term care. *The Gerontologist, 29,* 633–639.

Kane, R. A., Caplan, A. L., Freeman, I. C., Aroskar, M. A., & Urv-Wong, E. K. (1990). Avenues to appropriate autonomy: What next? In R. A. Kane & A. L. Caplan (Eds.), *Everyday ethics: Resolving dilemmas in nursing home life (pp. 306-317).* New York: Springer.

Kapp, M. A. (1989). Medical empowerment of the elderly. *Hasting Center Report, 19,* 5–7.

Lecso, P. A. (1989). Murder-suicide in Alzheimer's disease. *Journal of the American Geriatrics Society, 37,* 167–168.

Risks and Choices: When Is Paternalism Justified?

■

Carol A. Tauer

Several years ago, I participated in a conference sponsored by Adult Protection Services, State of Minnesota. The title of that conference was, "It's Good, But Is It Right?" We applied this question to each case we discussed, examining two aspects of each client's situation: What is in the best interests of this person, or what is *good* for him or her? And second, to what extent is it *right* to intervene to achieve that good in opposition to the person's preferences or choices?

The case study "Risky Business" raises the same issues. For each of the three clients in the case study, the case manager must make an assessment of needs and resources for meeting these needs to propose a plan that would be *good* for this client. But when the client has a differing view of the situation and expresses preferences that involve an element of risk, the case manager must decide whether to oppose the client's wishes. If the manager believes the client's needs are not adequately met by the arrangements the client wants or chooses, then the manager faces an ethical dilemma: To protect the health and safety of this client, is it *right* for me or my agency to override the client's wishes? (Young, Pignatello, & Taylor, 1988).

A basic ethical principle relating what is good to what is right is the principle of autonomy. According to the principle of autonomy, those who are capable of decision making must be allowed to make their own choices, even if they put themselves into situations that, in the judgment of others, may not be best for them (Buchanan, 1981). Autonomy has high priority as an ethical principle for two reasons: (a) the entire moral life rests on the assumption that each of us is a moral agent responsible for his or her own choices; and (b) each of us is the best judge of what is in our own best interests, because interests are closely related to personal values and preferences.

The weight given to autonomy as an ethical principle does not mean that it is absolute, however. Autonomy is limited by the resources that are available, and no one has a right to demand or expect more than a fair share of the community's resources. The case manager here plays the role of a gatekeeper in managing resources and ensuring a fair allocation of them (Kane, 1990). In the cases described in "Risky Business," the issue of limited resources lurks in the background, but it is not a central issue.

In these cases we are more concerned with other possible limitations on autonomy, primarily these two: A client may not be capable of the decision making that is required; or a client may be identifiable as a "vulnerable adult," a legal concept with ethical implications. Each of these conditions limits the client's autonomy, specifically his or her prerogative to choose situations that involve risks to personal well-being and safety.

A client who is not capable of decision making is often called "incompetent." "Incompetence" involves a legal determination and may not be the best category for sorting out those who are unable to make their own decisions. The President's Commission for the Study of Ethical Problems in Medicine (1982) used the term *decisional capacity*, and focused on the abilities actually needed to make health care or life care decisions.

The commission enunciated three characteristics that a person must have to make these decisions: a reasonably stable set of values and goals, the ability to understand information and to communicate in some way, and the ability to reason and deliberate about the options and their consequences (President's Commission, 1982). Assessment of decisional capacity does not require special professional expertise; a lay person, and certainly a trained case manager, should be able to make the assessment in most cases.

Because decisional capacity relates to the decisions that actually must be made, it is often described as "task specific" (see the commentary by Brody in chapter 6). A person may be able to make decisions in one area (e.g., living situation) but not in another (e.g., financial affairs). The level of understanding and deliberation required will vary from one task to another, depending on the complexity of the information and options (Annas & Densberger, 1984; Buchanan & Brock, 1989). Thus, an overall judgment of "competent" or "incompetent" provides too rough a classification. Similarly, the Mental Status Questionnaire, although perhaps useful for other purposes, is not designed to determine a client's ability to make the specific and practical decisions portrayed in "Risky Business."

The concept of "vulnerable adult," which is defined legally in many states, may entail limitations on a client's choice of risks even if the client has decisional capacity. The ethical basis for the legal requirement is the principle of justified paternalism: We are ethically obligated to protect those who are vulnerable, or in some way incapable of protecting or taking care of themselves.

A person is vulnerable when, although appearing to choose a particular arrangement or situation, he or she is really unable to make a voluntary choice. This person may be coerced by others (perhaps by a relative or caregiver), or could be coerced by internal pressures that diminish freedom, for example, by chemical dependency. This sort of vulnerability often requires intervention by the case manager, even if the client protests.

A person is also vulnerable when unable or unwilling to recognize and remedy serious threats to personal well-being. These threats include physical or sexual abuse by others, and failure or inability to care for basic needs: nutrition, warmth, hygiene, and essential health care. Such threats to the client's welfare are so serious that they limit the vulnerable client's right to choose to continue in such situations. But the threats must be actual problems at the present time, not simply a prediction that something like this might possibly happen in the future.

Let us now begin an examination of the three clients in "Risky Business." I will take them in reverse order, starting with Miss J, who cooperates with an adequate care plan and has no current problems, though she has a deteriorating illness. Miss J has told her case manager that she plans to kill herself when her condition deteriorates much further and that she hopes to avoid a nursing home at all costs.

Miss J's plan to commit suicide is not really a risk, but rather it is a choice. At the present time, there are no grounds for overriding her presumed wishes to remain in her own home. We have no information that suggests that her mind is deteriorating, or that she lacks the capacity to make her own decisions. Many people have a similar plan to end their own lives, given certain conditions (e.g., members of the Hemlock Society). The fact that Miss J's plan may reach its terminus sooner than that of someone in their forties or fifties, is not an adequate reason for acting more forcibly toward her. And as the National Rifle Association is fond of reminding us, she does have the same constitutional right to possess a gun as any other noncriminal does. Either to take the gun away from her, or to put her into protective custody because of a speculative threat, would be an unwarranted violation of her autonomy.

But these remarks do not imply that the case manager should simply "wash her hands" of the matter. There are alternatives that should be explored. One wonders why Miss J revealed her plan to the manager. Is Miss J asking for something? Some psychosocial support that is missing in her life? Some assurance that her antipathy to residence in a nursing home will be taken seriously when other arrangements for her care have to be made? Nevertheless, the case manager must be careful not to promise something that cannot be guaranteed, even in the hope of preventing a suicide. Perhaps the case manager should consider whether Miss J's care plan, while dealing admirably with her physical needs, is neglecting social, psychological, and spiritual needs that are also important to her.

Mr. K, the client in the second case, lives out in the country and "needs so much more care than [his care] program can offer." There is no evidence that he lacks the ability to understand his situation, or to choose it voluntarily. In fact, when he was in the hospital because of a broken hip, he exerted positive efforts to return to his home as soon as possible.

Because the written case does not provide much detail, it is difficult to get a good sense of the care needed by Mr. K that he is not receiving. The case suggests that his care is adequate only because kind and helpful neighbors supplement the services arranged by the case manager. The manager seems concerned that the neighbors may not continue their helpful efforts indefinitely, because it's not really their responsibility. Conversely, the manager considers *asking* them to stop helping to provoke a crisis.

If the neighbors are really willing to "pitch in" and take up the slack in helping Mr. K, I see no reason for discouraging them from doing so. Neighborly communities that care about their vulnerable members should be supported and encouraged, not made to feel as if they're out of line. However, it may be that the neighbors feel caught in this situation, would like to withdraw, and are even somewhat resentful of what they perceive to be an imposition. If this is the case, then the situation should be faced honestly; the case manger will have to explain to Mr. K that his neighbors can no longer play a major role in meeting his needs. But first, the case manager must find out what the neighbors' attitudes really are.

There appear to be two specific areas of concern to Mr. K's case manager. The first is a serious one; if he has an accident or becomes seriously ill, he might not be found for some time. (When he fractured his hip, he was not found for 19 hours.) This concern must be addressed, but surely there must be alternatives to moving Mr. K to another setting against his wishes. Perhaps he could wear a device that would enable him to signal in case of need, or perhaps a neighbor (even a preteen or teenager) could check his home on a regular basis. If he has a telephone, a system could be established for regular contact. Ingenuity is needed here.

The case manager's other concern is Mr. K's inability to bring in the wood necessary to heat his home next winter. To those of us who have financial resources, this seems like a small point; we would simply hire someone to bring in the wood. If there are no resources to pay for this service, either because it is not an allowed expense, or because (as seems the case) Mr. K has reached the limit of what can be expended on his care, then the matter should be discussed with Mr. K. What are his ideas? Would he prefer to have financial resources used for this service or for conversion to another type of heating rather than for something else he considers less essential? Is there room for some flexibility?

This case needs imagination and consultation, with Mr. K and with his neighbors, not an attempt to provoke an artificial crisis. A case manager who would provoke such a crisis risks doing more harm than good. By engaging in manipulation and dishonesty, the manager not only behaves unethically, but damages the client's trust, diminishes his or her self-respect, and harms all relationships involved. It is very difficult to imagine any case management situation in which such provocation could be acceptable and could be expected to have good consequences. Honest, face-to-face discussion of concerns and options, although probably more time-consuming, is really the only ethical and professional course of action.

The last case, that of Mrs. D, is the most complex one. Mrs. D's situation, more than the other two cases, may possibly satisfy criteria for justifiable limitations on client preferences. First, the case manager expresses uncertainty about the client's "competence," or her ability to make her own decisions about her living situation. However, no evidence is given for this uncertainty other than the suggestion that a "normal person" wouldn't want to live this way. Because "normal persons" choose a wide variety of life-styles, given the options available to them, this observation does not demonstrate Mrs. D's decisional incapacity. But if the case manager really has legitimate doubts, then she or someone else should do an assessment.

An assessment of Mrs. D's decision-making capacity should not rely on *what* she chooses, nor on her ability to perform a broad range of mental tasks. It must focus on her ability to make a decision about her care and her living situation, using a thought process that shows that she understands the facts, the advantages and disadvantages, the alternatives, and the future possible consequences. If she demonstrates awareness of these elements but, all things considered, still prefers her current situation, there is no reason to presume her choice should be invalidated.

It is possible that Mrs. D is able to understand her situation and its drawbacks, but is unable to choose it voluntarily. She may be under the influence of her caregiver to such an extent that she is unable to make a voluntary choice, or to see any other option as a real possibility. In Mrs. D's case, she is not coerced by the lack of other noninstitutional options, because her daughter would like to take her into her home. But psychologically, she may not be able to envision living anywhere else. Because there appears to be no specific or concrete coercion exercised by her caregiver, Mrs. D's own psychology may be the main coercive factor. To try to explore this possibility (e.g., through psychotherapy) seems pointless at this stage in Mrs. D's life. But the case manager should reassure herself that the caregiver is not making use of manipulative strategies that would be an external form of coercion and that would have to be dealt with.

Given the evidence provided in the written case, one would conclude that Mrs. D apparently is capable of deciding on her living arrangements and caregiver. But we still have to consider whether her vulnerability requires us to protect her against serious and immediate threats to her well-being. Is Mrs. D being abused, or perhaps not receiving adequate care for her basic needs?

The case manager suspects that Mrs. D is being exploited financially, that the caregiver and her family are cheating Mrs. D. Exploitation is a form of abuse. But besides the fact that this financial exploitation is unproven, it seems to be quite minor, even if true. As long as Mrs. D has adequate food, shelter, and nursing care, she may not be concerned about where a portion of her check goes. Or she may consider its loss as an informal compensation for care, without the embarrassment and hassle that formal payment arrangements between friends might involve. At the very least, the case manager should clarify the facts of this matter before she takes further steps.

A second element of exploitation might be found in the live-in arrangements for the caregiver's two sons. Here we are missing an important and highly relevant fact: Whose apartment is it? If it is the caregiver's and she pays the rent, then Mrs. D is hardly being exploited by the sons. If the apartment is Mrs. D's and she pays, then she is being exploited unless the sons pay rent to her. If Mrs. D and the caregiver share rent, then a negotiation is in order, and the sons should pay their share.

Apart from financial exploitation, it is difficult to see how the sons' presence harms Mrs. D. Their problems with the law and with drugs are vague and unproven. No behavioral traits that endanger Mrs. D are mentioned. The apartment may be a bit crowded, but, then again, Mrs. D may like having some young people around.

Mrs. D seems to be in good condition, which is particularly admirable in light of all the care she requires. The case study describes her care as "meticulous"; one wonders why the proposed discussion question cites a "less than adequate caregiver." We have no way of knowing that Mrs. D's daughter would do better—or whether the daughter has teenage or young adult children who might also have some difficulties in the growing up process.

The case manager needs to clarify many aspects of this case: Mrs. D's decisional capacity, whether the caregiver is coercing Mrs. D's decision, the truth about Mrs. D's checks, whether the caregivers' sons are living in Mrs. D's apartment free of charge, and Mrs. D's attitude toward the sons' presence. The manager's next move will depend on the answers to these questions. Coercion or clear exploitation on the part of the caregiver or her sons must be confronted. We cannot allow a vulnerable person to be coerced, or to choose to be exploited in any explicit or significant way. (Note that we all permit some interactions that could be identified as minor exploitations.)

But if Mrs. D is as mentally capable as she appears to be, is not being coerced, is not being "ripped off" financially, and is not being harmed by the sons, there seems to be no reason not to allow her to remain where she prefers to be.

Her daughter's frequent calls should be welcomed. She is taking seriously a responsibility that belongs to her. The case manager should continue to respect Mrs. D's wishes that details not be shared with the daughter. Although the case manager may not have the professional status of a health care provider or social worker, hence may not have a clear professional code of confidentiality, her agency must have such a code. The case manager is strongly obligated to respect the client confidentiality to which the agency has committed itself. The fact that the person requesting information about Mrs. D is her daughter does not lessen this obligation, because Mrs. D is capable of giving permission for release of information and has specifically refused release of details to her daughter.

The daughter should be encouraged to visit her mother and to keep in contact with her as much as possible. Above all, the case manager must remember that Mrs. D is the client, not Mrs. D's daughter. The fact that the daughter is concerned is in itself no reason for the manager to change her own approach to the case. If the daughter did raise a particular concern as a result of her own observations or her conversations with her mother, that would provide more data for the case manager's evaluation of the case. But expressions of concern in themselves should not lead the manager to be more paternalistic toward Mrs. D than would otherwise be appropriate and ethical.

REFERENCES

Annas, G. J., & Densberger, J. E. (1984). Competence to refuse medical treatment: Autonomy vs. paternalism. *Toledo Law Review,* *15,* 561-592.

Buchanan, A. E. (1981). Medical paternalism. In M. Cohen, T. Nagel, & T. Scanlon (Eds.), *Medicine and moral philosophy*. Princeton: Princeton University Press.

Buchanan, A. E., & Brock, D. W. (1989). *Deciding for others: The ethics of surrogate decision making*. New York: Cambridge University Press.

Kane, R. A. (1990). What Is Case Management Anyway? In R. A. Kane, K. Urv-Wong, & C. King (Eds.), *Case management: What is it anyway?* Minneapolis: University of Minnesota Long-Term Care Decisions Resource Center.

President's Commission for the Study of Ethical Problems in Medicine and Biomedical and Behavioral Research (1982). *Making health care decisions*. Washington, DC: U.S. Government Printing Office.

Young, A., Pignatello, C. H., & Taylor, M. B. (1988). Who's the Boss? Ethical Conflicts in Home Care. *Health Progress, 83,* 59-62.

VIEW FROM THE FIELD

Perspective From California

■

Patrick Murphy

My comment on the case, "Risky Business: Who Decides on What Risks," and the two commentaries, comes from the operational perspective of a state department with oversight responsibility for case management for frail older persons and functionally impaired adults. The perspective is derived from two programs specifically, the Multipurpose Senior Services Program (MSSP) and Linkages.

MSSP is a program serving older persons aged 65 and older who are Medicaid (Medi-Cal) eligible and whose level of frailty would meet certification for admittance to a skilled or intermediate care nursing home. This is a Medicaid-Waiver program that serves up to 6,000 persons, at any one time, at 22 sites for a total of 8,941 clients annually. Total funding for the program annually is $20.7 million—funds are 50% federal and 50% State General Fund match.

The other program, called Linkages, is funded from State General Funds and local resources and serves frail elderly and functionally impaired adults aged 18 years and older with health or social problems that if left unattended would create a risk of nursing home placement. Total funding for this program is $2.1 million and serves 75 or more clients at each of 13 sites.

All decisions, risky or otherwise, affecting the well-being of clients in these programs have to be made within the overall parameters, policies, and guidelines that govern each program. Examples of these controlling factors include compliance with contractual agreements, client eligibility criteria, level of client care determination, and the cost effectiveness of maintaining the client in the program. These issues we all know well. They are well defined and the standards relatively easy to reference.

The issues raised here, however, are not so easy to address. Before committing these comments to paper, I consulted with staff from the California Department of Aging and from selected local program sites. In most cases, staff was quite familiar with the issues raised by "Risky Business: Who Decides on What Risks," and their comments did not differ greatly from the commentators' viewpoints, although there were some exceptions.

On the issue of beneficence versus autonomy of the client, we identified an element of program structure which helps us deal with such problems. Our case-management program employs a multidisciplinary team approach to care planning which involves a health professional, a social worker and a supervisor. In this way, the programs provide a balanced and comprehensive treatment of all issues including beneficence or safety of the client, and the client's right to autonomy and self-determination. Generally, we endorse the view that autonomy of the client is reflective of all the rights of people in a free society and thus to be maximized as a primary goal of case management.

Regarding intervention by the case manager, the principles espoused by the commentators found wide acceptance and agreement among us. Interesting to me, however, was that in the case of Miss J, the suicide-leaning client with the gun. Our staff had general agreement with the comment that Miss J could be making a legitimate choice given that she possessed the capacity to do so, and that all alternatives had been explored. There was no support forthcoming for the point that the gun needed to be removed as a factor of immediate threat—although, personally I appreciated the point made regarding her immediate and long-range autonomy.

In the case of Mr. K, our staff gave no support for provoking a crisis to bring about a perceived good. In general, we felt that provoking a crisis for any reason is more of an emotional reaction rather than a well-planned strategy that is clearly developed and understood by both the case manager and the client.

In the case of Mrs. D, the case-management staff agreed that there was more conjecture than facts presented, and that a cost-benefit analysis would show that the financial loss was quite small in comparison with the benefit provided to Mrs. D.

There was vehement support for the point that we are too quick to abandon autonomy in the case of an older person, simply because they are older and may need assistance in certain areas.

In many instances in our experience, neither the client nor case manager makes the rules—others do this, for example, landlords or doctors. The case manager is seen as the interface between the client and society, and is often cast in the roles of buying time, defining issues, and exploring alternatives for the client. Quite often, by the time someone applies to our programs, their support system is already collapsing, and their families and other persons involved are close to burnout. The case manager's role then is to support the supports, advocate for the client within reason, provide counseling, and arrange respite. More direct intervention may be taken if the client is clearly a danger to self or others.

Our site directors impart to their case managers a philosophy that their primary goal is to maintain people in their own communities, and thus that person's right to self-determination must be upheld and supported. Case managers are advised not to substitute their judgment or value system for that of the client. Rather, through careful analysis and assessment, their mission is to determine and support the client's personal value system. Additional principles that characterize our programs include the following:

- No case manager need ever handle any case alone.
- The case manager always aims to identify the resources that optimize the client's control of their situation.
- The case manager clearly communicates the limits of case management, and as a result should not have to discontinue or initiate something precipitously.
- The case manager has an array of support tools and must know what each can and cannot do.
- The case manager's awareness that working with people who are at risk means there are going to be de facto risks involved.
- Recognition that the potential to do harm is always there by virtue of an intervention in someone's life.
- Because of the preceding, we hire people of caliber and qualifications, to whom we say, "use your judgment to do the least intervention necessary to get the job done."

EDITORS' QUESTIONS FOR FURTHER DISCUSSION

■

1. Are there any limits to the risks clients can choose to face?
2. Are there any limits to the risks that case managers must tolerate?
3. Is it ever ethical to provoke a crisis to improve the client's care?
4. Should the case manager's stance toward risk taking of the client change when family members raise concerns?
5. Are risks of deliberate self-harm (as in the cases of Miss J and Mrs. D) different from risks because the program can't provide enough care (as in Mr. K's case). And is the self-harm of someone who might plan a "rational suicide" different from the self-harm of Mrs. D, who puts up with a less than adequate caregiver?

Chapter 5

YOU WOULDN'T LEAVE A FIVE-YEAR-OLD ALONE: Care Plans That Do Right by Incompetent Clients

CASE

■

Case managers say that situations with dementia—diagnosed or undiagnosed, advanced or incipient—cause them the greatest moral dilemmas. These dilemmas are never clearcut. First of all, one has to decide whether the client is capable of decision making. And when the client isn't capable of decision making, then the case manager has to decide what to do with a thousand case details.

Mrs. R seems confused sometimes and sometimes is right on the button. She will laugh at your jokes and tell her own. The next time you see her, she won't remember who is in her family. The case manager knows Mrs. R really well because she has been monitoring the case for several years. She arranged for a homemaker and a bathing service for Mrs. R, who lives alone in a high-rise apartment. Now questions are being raised about her competence to continue in the apartment. One time she left the stove on and a small fire occurred. It wasn't a big deal—Mrs. R's worker arrived and put it out, but it could have been serious. Mrs. R was chagrined and decided that she would take her meals in the dining room and not do much cooking any more. Mrs. R's daughter isn't convinced that other problems won't occur and would like her mother in a safer situation. She has asked the doctor for an opinion. Mrs. R isn't about to turn over her affairs willingly. She thinks she can manage things quite well and likes her living situation. She is willing to have her son-in-law balance her checkbook but wants to retain the right to make all other decisions. Based on a half-hour consultation, the doctor says that Mrs. R is incompetent. The case manager doesn't think she's at that stage yet and thinks she is in a much better position to judge because of her long involvement. She wonders if she should make an issue of it.

Mrs. S, age 97, is definitely incompetent. She has Alzheimer's disease with moderately severe memory loss. Her behavior is socially appropriate and she is not disruptive, but she certainly could not anticipate dangers or take actions for her own safety in emergencies. She lives with her grandson, who works a 9-hour day. Mrs. S receives the maximum amount of services the program can give, which is 4 hours a day. She also receives care from her grandson and other family members, but Mrs. S is alone for as much as 4 to 5 hours at a stretch. Sometimes she is also alone at night when her grandson goes out.

The family is satisfied with this arrangement, even though they realize that Mrs. S may fall into harm. If Mrs. S dies at home, the relatives promise they will hold the agency blameless. They do lock her in the house because, all things considered, this seems safest. The stove has been adjusted and reasonable safety precautions taken. The family feels this is a better arrangement than a nursing home.

This is not as bad as last year's case where the daughter locked her mother in a barn for 8 hours at a time—that was malevolent, whereas here there is an effort to make the best of a bad situation in the interests of the family member. But, still, the case manager feels that she should not countenance Mrs. S's situation. The client is demented, after all, and cannot speak for herself. One would not leave a 5-year-old alone, nor would one lock him or her in a house. The case manager's choices are to keep working toward a nursing home placement, to accept the situation, or to withdraw entirely so as not to countenance an unsafe situation.

COMMENTARIES

Beyond the Double Agent:
Toward a Systemic Ethics of Case Management

■

Susan M. Wolf

It would be easy to assume case managers to be a species of the genus "caregiver," and so subject to the same kind of ethic that governs the doctor-patient relationship or other types of therapeutic caregiving. Thus one might begin to intone the familiar quartet of autonomy, beneficence, nonmaleficence, and justice (Beauchamp & Childress, 1989). Though there actually is no unitary caregiving ethic—one can find significant differences in the role and obligations of doctor, nurse, and respiratory therapist, for example—the quartet is usually used in some combination to describe the ethical obligations of each type of caregiver. The predictable (though often quite important) punch line is that the caregiver must honor the patient's or client's autonomy and arrange care accordingly.

One could analyze the cases of Mrs. R and Mrs. S in just this way. One could argue that the case manager holds the fate of a vulnerable and dependent person in her hands. Thus the case manager, like a doctor, could be seen as standing in a fiduciary relation to that person. One could then derive a duty for the case manager to protect and advocate. I present that analysis subsequently in what I hope are strong terms, approaching the ethics of case management as one type of therapeutic ethic. This analysis leads one to conclude that the case manager must place client service and advocacy first.

But I then go on to critique this analysis as wishful thinking at best and a danger to clients at worst. The conclusion may be proper, but given the realities of case management, the analysis is deeply flawed. It is not at all clear that case managers are really "like" physicians or other direct caregivers in relevant ways, and so bound by any version of a therapeutic ethic. Although many are nurses or social workers, many are not professionals governed by standards that transcend the terms of their employment (see chapter 2). Thus they may not be agents of the client at all, but of the agency or system of which they are a part. Indeed, much of the discussion of ethical problems faced by case managers hinges on seeing them as double agents, torn between serving the client's needs and the rules and needs of their agency or system (Dubler, 1992).

Finally, I go on to suggest how one might begin to construct a more defensible ethics of case management. One must recognize the ways in which case management is nested within a broader system. This suggests that the ethical obligations of case managers are to be found not in the fiction that they are professionals with independent obligations, but precisely in their functioning as a specific part of a system. Thus I argue that the system itself must operate within certain limits, providing substantive and procedural safeguards, and case managers have an important role to play within that framework. This suggests that pivotal entities are missing from the cases of Mrs. R and Mrs. S—the agency and broader system. Only when one's vision includes those players can one develop a defensible ethics for case management, what I will call a "systemic ethic." Then the problem of double agency is transformed. No longer is the case manager torn between equal claims to advocate for client and system. Instead, we recognize the truth—that the case manager is always part of the system. But we also recognize particular obligations toward the client because of that. It is this, then, that I am suggesting properly grounds arguments about the case manager's duties toward the client.

POSITION OF ARGUING FROM A THERAPEUTIC ETHIC

The argument from a therapeutic ethic begins with a recognition of the vulnerability of the client and the harm she risks suffering. The argument might look like the following:

Taking away an adult's control over her affairs, and compelling her to leave the home she knows and prefers, are among the most profound assaults one can visit on a person. These maneuvers, even when benignly motivated, radically interfere with a person's vision of her self and conduct of her life. Before a case manager instigates or participates in disenfranchising the adult and moving her, a heavy burden must be met, both in justifying these changes and in providing procedural protections for the individual so that she or her advocate may challenge the change.

The cases of Mrs. R and Mrs. S raise questions about whether that burden has been met and what the proper role of a case manager is when the "client" living at home is of questionable competence or clear incompetence, may be exposed to danger in remaining at home, but either wishes to remain or has a family who wishes it. I place the term "client" in quotes because one question raised by these cases is who the case manager's client really is and indeed whether she has a client at all. So the term here is used initially merely to designate the individual whose care and autonomy are centrally at issue.

The case of Mrs. R raises the question of whether a client's autonomy should be compromised on the basis of a physician's assessment that the person is incompetent. The case manager considers deferring to a supposedly medical assessment of incompetence, with the implication that Mrs. R will then be removed from the home she prefers and deprived of control over her affairs. Yet the facts of the case indicate that the physician's assessment merits challenge, not deference. The case manager should mount a challenge because the assessment seems factually wrong and professionally substandard, the case manager seems to be the only one available to mount any challenge, and if the case manager has *any* duties of advocacy to Mrs. R those duties would have to include preventing error and harm. Finally, the danger to Mrs. R seems not so great as to seriously ground an argument for overriding her preferences.

The physician's global assessment that Mrs. R is incompetent appears flawed and substandard for several reasons (Buchanan & Brock, 1989). First, "incompetence" is an assessment only a court can make, according the person due process protections before taking the drastic step of disenfranchising them. Nonjudicial professionals only assess decisional capacity. Second, there is widespread agreement that capacity is not all or nothing; it can fluctuate. That appears to be the case here, with Mrs. R sometimes fully oriented and sometimes not. There is also widespread agreement that capacity is most properly conceived as decision specific. A person may no longer be able to balance her checkbook but may well be able to care for herself in the home. Thus the physician's global assessment of Mrs. R's "incompetence" seems uninformed both by the facts and the most relevant thinking about the nature of capacity.

Even if Mrs. R demonstrated a greater lack of capacity than shown here, that itself would not be enough to violate her wishes concerning placement and control over her own activities. It is widely agreed that respect for individual autonomy demands not only respect for the current wishes of persons with capacity and respect for the past wishes of persons who previously had capacity, but also consideration of the current wishes of persons who have lost capacity. An adult who has lived a life, developing values and preferences, and who can still communicate what actions would be consistent with those values or preferences deserves to be heard and to have her values and preferences govern to the greatest possible extent. An adult who has lost capacity is not the equivalent of a 5-year-old who has never had it.

Thus the case manager has not only the option to challenge the physician's pronouncement but also the duty to do so. The physician's pronouncement dresses up in medical language an unnuanced and uninformed judgment about Mrs. R's capacities. It also provides inadequate ethical grounds for overriding Mrs. R's wishes and depriving her of control over her affairs. Mere incapacity to make a certain set of decisions only implies that someone else—typically, some sort of surrogate—should take over the decisional authority. The surrogate is supposed to continue guiding the decisions in accordance with the person's preferences. Thus, incapacity itself would not mean that Mrs. R should be forced to leave her home. To question seriously continued deference to her wishes, there would have to be such grave threat to her health, safety, and well-being as to indicate that she herself would opt for a safer setting if she could fully appreciate the relevant factors.

The case manager is also obligated to challenge the physician if the case manager conceives of Mrs. R as her client in any robust sense. If the manager owes allegiance to Mrs. R as a client, then she must advocate in accordance with Mrs. R's wishes. She must also protect Mrs. R's rights and interests by providing, through that challenge, procedural protection for Mrs. R. At the very least, those procedural protectors should take the form of requiring full explanation from the physician, questioning the appropriateness of the physician's assessment, and resisting resulting actions that would compromise Mrs. R's wishes, rights, and interests.

Only this kind of single-minded advocacy for Mrs. R makes the use of the term "client" appropriate. The dictionary reveals that the term derives from the Latin "cliens," meaning "dependent, follower" (American Heritage, 1980). A client is one who depends on the more expert professional to act *for* her. Only if the manager responds as a fiduciary to Mrs. R's dependency and advocates for her is the language of "client" defensible. Some might argue that the entire family is the client here. But this is incoherent. When a family is divided, as in this case, one cannot act *for* more than one of the warring parties at once.

This still leaves the question of whether the case manager *should* seek a true client relationship with Mrs. R. After all, the manager's role is a tricky one, because she also acts as gatekeeper to certain resources, a function in tension with the advocacy role. One can argue, however, that the manager should indeed press herself into the role of individual client advocate. The most compelling argument is that *someone* must play that role to protect Mrs. R and her rights and interests, and no one else is doing it. Based on similar logic, one can argue that in the acute care setting a patient's primary physician should act as her advocate even though the physician also performs a gatekeeping function controlling the patient's access to certain health care resources. Indeed, one can maintain that in both settings the professional's decisions about access should be guided by the duty of advocacy.

In contrast to Mrs. R, Mrs. S has definitely lost capacity. It is unclear what Mrs. S's previous wishes were, or indeed whether she is even still living in a setting she has known and loved. Nonetheless, her family wishes her to remain in the grandson's home. It is not clear why. The case describes the burdens and dangers to Mrs. S—she is locked in the house alone for hours at a stretch, and would be unable to respond to an emergency if one arose—but does not give a full picture of the pros and cons of the alternative possible settings including the current one.

Here it would seem that the case manager's first obligation is to discover more facts. The manager must do this to be able to advocate for Mrs. S's past wishes and values, if they can be ascertained from the family. If Mrs. S's wishes and values cannot be ascertained, then the manager will need more facts anyway to judge what setting would be in Mrs. S's best interests.

This is a case in which it is even more important to clarify who the client is than it was in the prior case. The family is so eager to retain the current arrangement that they offer to hold the agency blameless even if Mrs. S dies. But the family cannot relieve the manager of her professional obligations to serve Mrs. S in a way that is ethical and comports with professional obligations of due care.

Mrs. S's case manager is rightly distressed, because the family is trying to dissuade her from serving Mrs. S, whose situation requires investigation. But the case manager must beware of the shape her distress is taking—analogizing Mrs. S to a 5-year old. Mrs. S is not a 5-year old. She is an adult with prior capacity, who lived a life in which she established certain values and preferences. The case manager must uncover those values and preferences, and then work with everyone involved to permit those values and preferences to guide the fate of Mrs. S.

Critique

The form of the argument above should be familiar. In essence, it is the same type of argument often used to make sense of the ethical obligations of a physician or other caregiver. There are a couple of points added to deal with some of the idiosyncracies of case management—use of the term "client" instead of "patient," an occasionally exhortatory tone because of the ethical uncertainties still besetting case management, and the plea that *someone* must act for the client. But the argument generally proceeds by treating case management as a professional calling subject to yet another version of the familiar therapeutic ethic.

There are basically four strategies the argument uses to fit case management into the therapeutic ethic—four cornerstones, if you will, to the ethical structure built. First, the argument focuses on the fact that the clients are vulnerable, at risk, and in need of assistance and advocacy. The case manager, with greater knowledge of available resources and power over them than the client, can either help or hurt. Given the client's dependency, exposure, and disadvantage, the argument casts the case manager as a fiduciary with obligations to do good for the client and refrain from hurting her.

The first strategy is supported by a second—the use of the language of "client." Although the argument pauses to defend the word, it does so by once again focusing on the dependency and needs of that person. It does not ask whether the person on the other side of the relationship—the case manager herself—fulfills the requirements of the correlative role of "professional." After all, many of us encounter dependent, "following" people all the time whether it be our children, our elderly parents, or someone who has just slipped and fallen in the street. Yet none of those people become our clients simply by virtue of their dependency. Indeed, they do not become our clients unless we approach them in the role of a professional. The preceding analysis never looks carefully at this question in analyzing the role of the case manager. It simply allows the terminology of "client" to conjure up an implied vision of the case manager as a professional serving this vulnerable person.

The third argumentative strategy used is to argue by means of elimination. Beginning from the fact that no one else is protecting the client and advocating for her, the argument spots the case manager as a likely candidate for the role. The analogy to the doctor-patient relationship is lurking here. Because it is so commonplace to argue that every patient must have a primary physician managing her care and looking out for her, the argument seeks an analogous person to serve Mrs. R and Mrs. S, and so casts the case manager. There is no serious consideration given to the fact that maybe the case manager cannot serve that role, that perhaps she cannot resolve the advocate-gatekeeper double-agency bind the way the argument claims a physician might. The argument does not contemplate the possibility that as the situation is set up, there may be no one who can truly advocate for the client.

The fourth argument is a related argument from desperation. The physician in the case of Mrs. R seems to have made a mistake in assessing competence. The argument summons the case manager to challenge the physician and set wrong to right. Thus the strategy is to arm the case manager with the expertise, authority, and mission to take on the doctor. The argument depicts the case manager as a professional who is subject to a therapeutic ethic, because the only other professional in the picture—one who *is* subject to a therapeutic ethic—is failing.

All of these strategies for applying the familiar therapeutic ethic to case management are profoundly flawed. First of all, they underestimate the degree of uncertainty that still surrounds the role of case manager. Case managers operate in a variety of systems, paid by different masters, and subject to different rules. It may be that at this point in time there is no gelled, single role we can neatly label "case manager." Thus an adequate ethical analysis might have to seek much more information than given by these cases to figure out what kind of case manager we are talking about in what kind of system.

What we might find out could thoroughly disrupt the analogy to other caregivers. We might find out that the rules and ethos of the system within which the case manager operates leave her very little room to accommodate the wishes of the vulnerable person. Thus the first cornerstone would crumble. Yes, the "client" is vulnerable and at risk, but the case manager is not in a position or of a mind to serve her.

Similarly, the second cornerstone is shaky. We learn from empirical work that many case managers may not be professionals at all. Thus they may not be part of any group showing the hallmarks of a profession—specialized expertise, professional autonomy, and obedience to the standards of one's peers. Instead, case managers may simply be employees subject to the rules set by their agency or employer. If so, the language of "client" is self-delusion at best. The case manager is not a professional who is bound to challenge the employer who seeks a deviation from professional standards; the manager is an employee seeking to keep her job. She is in no position to serve a "client" with the necessary professionalism and independence. At worst, the language of "client" is a danger. It suggests to the vulnerable person that she has an advocate, serving her with independence and without conflict. Yet that is not the case.

The arguments by elimination and from desperation will not save the day. They cannot ground application of a therapeutic ethic. Instead, they simply point out the terrible fact that no one is truly serving the client. The therapeutic ethic is only wishful thinking.

MOVEMENT TOWARD A SYSTEMIC ETHICS OF CASE MANAGEMENT

One cannot create an ethics for case management by ignoring the obvious. Case managers typically are employees operating as part of a broader system. Indeed, the focus of this book is on publicly subsidized case management. Thus we are essentially talking about governmental employees—bureaucrats who operate as a small piece of a bigger system. We cannot pretend that these are independent caregivers who can simply ignore the terms of their employment and rules of their agency. Nor can we pretend that case managers are professionals who can or would claim that they are subject to independent standards of care, and so can base resistance to their agency or employer on those standards.

One also cannot base an ethics for case management on a requirement of heroism. If case managers are really government workers playing by governmental or agency rules, the ethics of case management cannot routinely require heroic defiance of those rules. We have to assume case managers will instead act in keeping with those rules.

The key to establishing any plausible ethic here is accepting that case managers are indeed following the rules, and largely staying within the parameters set by the system. Thus the focus shifts to the system itself. We begin to query the contours and procedures of that system. What goals does it serve? To what extent does it serve the wishes of individual clients? To what extent does it not? How are the roles of different players within the system differentiated? Does anyone—the case manager or someone else—have the assigned role of advocating for the client to assure fairness and effective, high-quality care? Or is no one really serving that function in a whole-hearted way? Is all of this disclosed to the client? Or is the client led to believe that the case manager (or someone else) is her advocate, when that is really not the case?

These are the questions of systems design that leap to the fore, and should be the focus of much more work. There is actually a helpful and analogous literature already developed in the law. This literature looks at the structure of different procedural systems and the values they serve (Cover & Fiss, 1979). Thus one can ask to what extent does a system and set of rules protect the vulnerable patient or client, provide an advocate for her, demonstrate respect for her, and achieve fairness.

To examine the ethics of the system's design and rules does not absolve individuals who operate within that system of ethical obligations. First of all, a "system" does not design itself. There are people who do so, and who are ultimately responsible for its characteristics. Second, even after the system is designed, individual players will still be responsible for fulfillment of their roles, and for their exercise of discretion because the rules are unlikely to resolve all questions. Thus a "systemic ethic" will still place moral responsibilities on individuals.

Then what will the content of this systemic ethic be? The real challenge will be to devise an ethic that builds in a duty of advocacy for and protection of clients. A new version of some of the arguments that cropped up earlier in applying the therapeutic ethic can be used to justify building this duty into the systemic ethic—the fact that the client alone cannot understand and manipulate the system, the dearth of people fulfilling an advocacy function, and the client's vulnerability to mistake and substandard care unless there is an advocate. Switching from a one-on-one therapeutic ethic to a vision of the entire system makes creating a duty of advocacy both harder and easier. It is harder because you are asking the system to build in its own gadfly or trouble-maker—someone who will advocate for the client. But it is easier because you can design the system to accommodate an advocate, much as the criminal law system revolves around the central requirement of advocacy for the accused defendant but is still capable of ruling against some defendants.

Thus a systemic ethic could dictate the same ultimate conclusions about the cases of Mrs. R and Mrs. S as the therapeutic ethic, but would reach those conclusions by a different route. It would address first the design and mandates of the systems responding to these clients, and then the case managers' role within those systems. Indeed, a systemic ethic that took seriously the duty of client advocacy and assigned it to the case manager would demand more of the case manager than the therapeutic ethic. The case manager would have to disclose fully to the client her role in the system, the rules applicable to the client's circumstance, the extent to which the case manager could advocate for the client, and her conflicts in pursuing an advocacy role. Moreover, there would be less reason in the systemic approach to allow a case manager to fulfill conflicting roles. Instead, the roles would more likely be divided between different individuals, so that the case manager could be a true advocate for the client. Certainly we would not tolerate her presenting herself to the client as an advocate, while secretly juggling conflicting roles.

It is worth anticipating one important objection. The problem with developing a systemic ethic and approaching the problems of case management from within that ethic is that it seems to eliminate an independent point *outside* the system from which the case manager can critique and manipulate that system. This is a serious challenge, because some systems may indeed turn out to be unethical in design or operation. Yet it is an illusion to maintain that case managers right now occupy any such independent point; that was the thrust of my argument that they are most accountable to agency rules rather than independent professional standards. Then the question is how to foster systemic critique and create a standpoint from which to assess a system. The answer must lie in beginning to compare systems and develop standards by which to judge them. We need to create the vocabulary for and actual practice of critique. Only then can case managers and others assert that their system is poorly designed or functioning badly compared with other systems and systemic standards.

The heading of this section is "Movement Toward a Systemic Ethics of Case Management." The argument for a systemic ethic can only point the direction in which to move. There then remains the hard work of fleshing out the details of that ethic—the substantive commitments and procedural standards to which systems will be held. My plea for true advocacy within the system fills in a piece of the puzzle, but only a piece. Filling in the full picture will be much more complex.

Yet that complexity is unavoidable. The attempt to apply a more familiar therapeutic ethic mischaracterizes who case managers really are and ignores the rest of the puzzle. No plausible ethic can grow in such soil. We must move beyond such distortions and easy answers. Only an honest assessment of the full picture will really do.

REFERENCES

Beauchamp, T. L., & Childress, J. F. (1989). *Principles of biomedical ethics* (3rd ed.). New York: Oxford University Press.

Buchanan, A. E., & Brock, D. W. (1989). *Deciding for others: The ethics of surrogate decision making.* New York: Cambridge University Press.

The American Heritage dictionary of the English language (New College ed.). (1980). Boston: Houghton Mifflin.

Cover, R. M., & Fiss, O. M. (1979). *The structure of procedure.* Mineola, NY: Foundation Press.

Dubler, N. N. (1992). Individual advocacy as a governing principle. *Journal of Case Management, 1,* 82–86.

Clinical Determination of Competency and Existential Advocacy

■

Muriel B. Ryden

CASE OF MRS. R

Who Knows?

Uncertainty as to Mrs. R's mental status appears to be a predominant theme in this situation. The data provided are vague and imprecise. To say she is "confused" is not a useful clinical judgment. Confusion is an imprecise term that may irresponsibly label an elder (Wolanin & Phillips, 1981). Mrs. R is described as being "sometimes right on the button." However, the example that follows, "She'll laugh at your jokes and tell her own," is not necessarily an indicator of competency.

The fact that at times she does not remember "who all is in her family" suggests some memory loss. One incident is mentioned in which Mrs. R left the stove on. This by itself would not trigger questions about her competency if she were a younger person. Her response to that incident suggests that she possesses some insight and judgment. She was chagrined and she decided that she would take her meals in the dining room and not do much cooking any more. Another possible indication of good judgment and recognition of her own limitations is her willingness to have her son-in-law balance her checkbook.

Good ethical decisions require sound clinical information. A thorough assessment needs to be made of Mrs. R's mental status before conclusions can be drawn about her capability to make her own decisions about where and how to live.

Safety Versus Autonomy

Although her mental status is somewhat ambiguous, Mrs. R's desire for maintaining her own autonomy is clear. She wants to retain the right to make decisions and isn't about to turn over her affairs willingly. She likes her living situation. It appears that there is some concern on the part of her daughter as to whether or not Mrs. R is accurate in her perception that she can manage things quite well in her high-rise apartment. No additional data are provided as to why her daughter thinks that Mrs. R should be in a safer situation. The recurring conflict in the care of the aged between safety and autonomy surfaces here. The daughter is not convinced that "other problems won't occur." In valuing safety, and trying to protect vulnerable elderly from physical trauma, we sometimes mistakenly think it is possible to eliminate for them all of the everyday risks of human life we accept for ourselves. The hazards of possible falls, fire, and other projected dangers are more clearly seen than the less concrete costs of insulating the elder from threat—the loss of autonomy, the stifling experience of overprotection, the damage to self-esteem, and the uprootedness and transition shock of a move to a strange, but supposedly safe, environment.

Yet autonomy in deciding how much risk is acceptable rests on the triad of informed consent: access to information, voluntariness, and competence (Lynn, 1983). If Mrs. R were to be found to be clearly incompetent to decide her living arrangements, then the principle of beneficence takes priority over the principle of autonomy. Her daughter, the case manager and the physician then are faced with determining what is in her best interest.

What Else Is Going On?

The case situation does not make clear whether factors other than concern for her mother's safety also may be influencing the daughter's actions. No data are provided as to the amount of time and energy the daughter expends to assist her mother in living alone in her apartment. Her obligations to her own family may conflict with her sense of duty toward her mother. Is she pressuring for a move to assuage her own anticipated guilt if something happened? Is she concerned about what others think about her mother living alone? What has been the history of their relationship? What does the daughter envision as "a safer situation"? Assisted living? A nursing home? A move to live with the daughter or someone else? Nevertheless, whatever her motivation, the daughter does seek professional help. She has asked the physician for "an opinion." The case manager needs to understand the daughter's position in this situation. However, it is Mrs. R who is her client, not Mrs. R's daughter.

Word From the "Pros"

The two health care professionals in this situation—the doctor and the case manager—appear to differ in their assessment of Mrs. R's competency. The adequacy of the assessment and the accuracy of the conclusions each has made about Mrs. R's decisional capacity are not clear. Based on a half-hour consultation, the doctor says that Mrs. R is incompetent. The nature of his assessment and the data on which he made this conclusion are not provided. The duration of his relationship with Mrs. R is unknown.

We are told that the case manager knows Mrs. R "really well," because she has been monitoring the case for several years. The case manager disagrees with the doctor's conclusion, and "doesn't think she's at that stage yet." Because mental status is an important variable to be considered in case management, one would expect that the case manager has systematically assessed Mrs. R's mental status with a reliable and valid instrument over these years, but no such information is provided. Nevertheless, the knowledge gained from observing Mrs. R's patterns of behavior and changes over time, as well as the benefit of having seen her function within her own environment give the case manager important information that needs to be shared with the client, the daughter, and the physician in the decision-making process.

The doctor has said Mrs. R is incompetent. What is competence? The President's Commission for the Study of Ethical Problems in Medicine and Biomedical and Behavioral Research suggests that the term *decisional capacity* may be preferable. Questions about decisional capacity are usually raised only when clients choose a course of action different from what the physician or family consider to be in their best interest. Mental status, which is assessed in determining decisional capacity, is a multifaceted construct including level of consciousness, attention, orientation, language, memory, judgment, reasoning, and calculation (Kiernan, Mueller, Langston, & Van Dyke, 1987). In what sense is Mrs. R "incompetent"? Incompetent for what? Drane (1985) suggests that a sliding scale of competence may be useful in preference to one ideal competency test.

The slippery issue of "what is competence and how do you assess it?" is not the only factor to be considered in resolving the difference of opinion between case manager and physician. Turf and status issues also may play a part. The qualifications of the physician and the level of his or her awareness of issues related to care of the elderly are not known. No information is given as to the extent of the doctor's prior knowledge of Mrs. R and her situation. Have the case manager and the doctor established a prior working relationship? What is the level of collegial trust and respect between them? Does the discipline of the case manager (nursing or social work) make a difference? Does the gender of the two health care professionals affect their interaction as a team? Is the case manager assertive, self-assured, and articulate about her observations and conclusions?

Rest Four-Component Model of Moral Action

This situation closes with the case manager wondering if she should make an issue of her differing perspective. Her conflict may be illuminated by examining the four-component model of moral action articulated by Rest (1986). The first component, moral sensitivity, has already been demonstrated by the case manager, when she presented this situation as an example of ethical concerns related to practice. She was aware of ethical conflict in the case of Mrs. R. Moral reasoning, what *ought* to be done, and why, is the second component of the model. Details of the case manager's reasoning are lacking, and her moral position is not clearly articulated. Nevertheless, it is apparent that she views Mrs. R's situation differently from that of the daughter and the physician and seems to be weighing the possibility of acting as Mrs. R's advocate. She probably is wrestling with competing values: She may not only be concerned for Mrs. R's autonomy, but also perhaps values her relationship with the physician, and may not want to "rock the boat" by disagreeing; perhaps she also feels a need to conserve her own limited energy in a stressful work situation. This is the essence of Rest's third component, moral commitment, where the priority given to competing values determines whether moral action, the fourth component, is taken. We do not know whether the case manager took moral action and actually did what she thought she ought to do. Caring, ego strength, assertiveness, and interpersonal skills in conflict resolution all contribute to taking moral action.

Summary

In the best interests of the client, the doctor and the case manager have an obligation to provide the most accurate clinical information possible about Mrs. R's mental status. (Her physical health status does not appear to be a concern.) However, information giving alone is inadequate. Gadow (1980) suggests that such a consumer approach to clients in health care is seriously flawed. At the opposite end of the continuum from consumerism Gadow places paternalism, which in the past has been pervasive in health care, but which has been found frequently to be ethically bankrupt. Gadow describes the need for an approach she calls "existential advocacy" for clients. For Mrs. R and her daughter, this would mean having sound information as a basis. But it would mean facilitating authentic decision making by assisting Mrs. R and her daughter to clarify their own values. Existential advocacy would mean helping them determine their priorities when concerns about safety and autonomy conflict. The daughter may need to be challenged to look at the burdens as well as the benefits of safe settings for her mother. Mrs. R and her mother may require help in exploring possible alternative arrangements that represent some compromise.

CASE OF MRS. R

Process of Watching Grandma

Mrs. S is clearly incompetent, according to the information provided. The predominant concern in this situation appears to be the degree of supervision necessary for her well-being because she is described as unable to anticipate dangers or take actions for her own safety in emergencies. There is no evidence that she presents any threat to others, as her behavior is described as socially appropriate and not disruptive.

In contrast to Mrs. R's daughter, the family of Mrs. S appears less concerned with her safety and more concerned with keeping her out of a nursing home. They lock her in the house, apparently out of fear that her going outside would be hazardous, and they have adjusted the stove and taken "reasonable safety precautions." However, the family is willing to keep her locked in the house with no supervision for 4 to 5 hours at a time, even though they realize that she may "fall into harm," rather than to place her in an institution.

Issues of Autonomy

No references are made as to what Mrs. S wishes. Even though she is described as having moderately severe memory loss, that does not necessarily mean that she cannot speak for herself. An exploration of the degree to which she can express her own values and a discussion with the family of her previously articulated preferences would be desirable so that, to the extent possible, decisions can be made that respect her autonomy. What evidence is there of how would she have weighed the benefits versus the risks in this situation?

The rights of a family to be self-determining regarding the care and treatment of an incompetent family member have a strong tradition in this country, whether the individual in question is a child or an elder. For a social service agency successfully to override such rights would, in all likelihood, require clear and convincing evidence to the courts that the individual is in danger, or presents a threat to others. Perhaps creative problem solving by the case manager and family might result in some strategies to provide more consistent supervision of Mrs. S.

What Constitutes Abuse and Neglect?

If a family can be prosecuted for abuse and neglect for leaving a 5-year-old child alone for hours in a locked house should similar treatment of an elderly family member who is cognitively impaired be considered abuse of a vulnerable adult? The family rejects the analogy, but their rationale is not given. The Minnesota law regarding reporting of maltreatment of vulnerable adults mandates reporting "abuse or neglect of a person who is unable or unlikely to report such abuse or neglect without assistance because of impairment of mental or physical function or emotional status" (Minnesota Statute 626.557). Failure by a caretaker to supply a vulnerable adult with necessary supervision is defined as neglect in this legislation.

What is "necessary supervision" for Mrs. R? Is it the same as for a 5-year-old? How does the cognitive function of an adult who apparently once was intact but now has moderately severe memory loss compare with the immaturely developed cognitive function of a 5-year-old? Do cognitively impaired adults retain a protective effect from previously well-learned patterns of behavior that children never have possessed? Mrs. S may have fluctuating mental function, which often is characteristic in this population. The extent to which Mrs. R's judgment is impaired may be equally or more important than the degree of her memory loss in assessing the hazards of leaving her alone in a locked house.

The family's motivation for keeping her in this situation is not clear. Who are the other family members besides the grandson? Who is making the decisions? Are they a caring family? What is their thinking? Why do they consider this to be a better arrangement than a nursing home? Are they attempting to honor her wishes? Do they think this situation is in her best interest? Is there an economic concern about not using up Mrs. S's resources to preserve an inheritance for the family?

Issues of Beneficence and Justice

Compassionate reasoning about what is the right thing to do in the provision of long-term care for cognitively impaired elderly in the community may require a reordering of the principles that have taken preemininence in the acute care setting. The advocacy role of supporting client autonomy may lessen as the client's ability to make informed decisions diminishes and be replaced with advocacy for beneficence— that is, for what is in the client's best interest. Attempts to honor advance directives as to living arrangements ("I never want to go to a nursing home") may flounder in the face of the reality of available options. Case managers have to consider what can reasonably be expected of the informal caregivers who may have conflicting obligations (Collopy, Dubler, & Zuckerman, 1990).

Issues of justice also influence case managers in their gatekeeping role and make them accountable to those beyond the client and family. To allocate fairly the social resources of the agency and the general public among competing claimants is an enormous challenge. For example, Mrs. R is receiving the maximum allowable number of hours of service.

Ideally, providing more services might solve the problem of supervision of Mrs. R when family members are absent, but this would deprive others of their share of agency services.

To continue to provide services in a situation in which the case manager believes the client is at risk may be considered "countenancing an unsafe situation." This may put the provider or the service agency at risk for liability. The case manager must wrestle with the question of whether it is more ethical to report the family and withdraw services (which might increase the amount of unsupervised time), or to continue services while attempting to convince the family that some alternative solution is necessary and possible.

REFERENCES

Collopy, B., Dubler, N., & Zuckerman, C. (1990). The ethics of home care: Autonomy and accommodation. *Hastings Center Report, 20* (Special Suppl.), 1–16.

Drane, J. (1985). The many faces of competency. *The Hastings Center Report, 15,* 17–20.

Gadow, S. (1980). Existential advocacy: Philosophical foundation of nursing. In S. F. Spiker & S. Gadow (Eds.), *Nursing: Images and ideas. Opening dialogue with the humanities* (pp. 79–101), New York: Springer.

Kiernan, R., Mueller, J., Langston, J. W., & Van Dyek, C. (1987). The neurobehavioral cognitive status examination: A brief but differentiated approach to cognitive assessment. *Annals of Internal Medicine, 107,* 481–485.

Lynn, J. (1983). Informed consent: An overview. *Behavioral Sciences and the Law, 1,* 29–45.

Minnesota Statute 6a26.557. Reporting of maltreatment of vulnerable adults.

Rest, J. R. (1986). *Moral development: Advances in research and theory.* New York: Praeger.

Wolanin, M. O., & Phillips, L. R. F. (1981). *Confusion: Prevention and care.* St. Louis: Mosby.

VIEWS FROM THE FIELD

Perspective from Minnesota

■

Todd Monson

These two case commentaries nicely illustrate that case management remains an art that lacks a written body of work to provide guidance regarding settled practices and norms for difficult cases. In the current state of case management, it is likely that different case management agencies and even different case managers within a single agency would often treat these situations differently.

SITUATION OF MRS. R

This is first and foremost a matter of public health and safety. Mrs. R lives in a high-rise apartment, she has some problems with cleaning and bathing, and she has already had one stove-top fire. It is one thing to live in a free-standing home and risk fires, but it is quite another to subject other people in the same building to harm. In fact I was surprised that there was no mention in the case summary of the building manager's response to the fire. Many buildings have policies that a resident's lease can be terminated when a resident endangers others.

The other major issue is that the client's physician has declared the client to be incompetent, but the case manager disagrees and is uncertain about challenging the physician's judgment. In my opinion, the case manager does need to ask the physician about the basis for the incompetency finding, but the physician's finding is not necessarily pivotal unless the physician proceeds to petition for an involuntary institutional placement. In addition the case manager does, I believe, need to help the client and family find a better living arrangement.

Mrs. R is clearly on the edge of independent living because she has demonstrated unsafe behavior. But the next change isn't necessarily to place Mrs. R in a nursing home. Although Mrs. R has some problems with short-term memory loss, it seems extreme to judge her unable to make decisions. In fact, she might do quite nicely in an assisted-living project or foster home, which would provide more monitoring. One assisted-living site manager told me that in her 5 years of work, she had never needed to terminate a client because of "unsafe" behavior.

The next step in the care planning process should be a care conference at which the building manager, the case manager, the daughter, the client, and the doctor "massage" the dilemma. There are a number of written guidelines for considering ethical dilemmas that the people at the care conference can use. Ultimately, Mrs. R and her daughter should receive ideas about some reasonable options from the care conference.

Mrs. R's situation is an excellent example of the need for a practical tool to help case managers differentiate an elderly person's ability to make decisions from a more general measure of cognitive impairment. At a recent conference on assessing decision-making capacity, Dr. Steven Miles posed an interesting delineation of three types of decisional ability: cognition, competence, and decision-making capacity. The last type, decision-making capacity, is very intriguing, but unfortunately I have not seen it used in a clinical setting (Miles, 1990). Currently many case managers and physicians rely on a measure of cognitive competence as proxy of decisional competence, but this is far from ideal. There are numerous examples of clients with moderate cognitive impairment who can and do make important decisions in specific circumstances.

CASE OF MRS. S

In reading about Mrs. S, age 97 with probable Alzheimer's disease, my first reaction was to wonder which of the "4 G's" was motivating her family to keep her at home yet leave her alone for extended periods—greed, gratitude, guilt, or agape. Beyond that, it seems to me that the case manager is faced with the quintessential dilemma about defining the client—is the family or Mrs. S the client? I believe that Mrs. S is the client, though the family obviously plays a pivotal role in her care.

One of the key issues in this case is the family's insight into the risk to which Mrs. S is being subjected. In other words, the family members should be able to articulate clearly their considerations of the following:

1. *Familiar environment*: Has Mrs. S lived for a long time in her current home or did she move in recently?
2. *Use of telephone:* Can Mrs. S dial 911 for help in an emergency?
3. *Physical safety*: Does Mrs. S frequently open the door to strangers?

Generally I believe that it is inappropriate to leave an incompetent person at home alone regularly for 4 to 5 hours if the person cannot dial 911 or often lets strangers in the house. If this is true in Mrs. S's case, I believe that the case manager should convene a care conference. If the family at that conference refuses to limit the time that the client is left alone, then the case manager should withdraw and refer the case to the local adult protection unit. In taking this action, the case manager is not forcing the client into a nursing home but rather is refusing to support a situation that in the case manager's professional judgment poses unreasonable risks for the client.

As is often the case in community-based long-term care, problems seem to be caused more by the family or caregivers than the client's specific behavior. In cases similar to this one, we have encountered families who simply refuse to compromise their beliefs that severe cognitively impaired people can be left alone for long periods. These same family members also have refused to accept services such as adult day care, which would reduce the time of being alone to a more reasonable length of time—for example, 1 to 2 hours.

Now I can hear some people saying "but, but, but. . . ." Nevertheless, without a base of hard data about the probabilities of harm occurring, I believe that case managers should not be forced to support a situation that in their own professional judgment (supported by other stakeholders) is unsafe. Perhaps we will someday be able to speak in a stochastic sense about the potential of a demented person being harmed when left alone. But until some clever soul gives us that information, we will need to use a very large dose of professional judgment in making our decisions.

REFERENCES

Miles, S. H. (1990). Assessing Decisional Capacity. In R. A. Kane, & C. D. King (Eds.), *Deciding whether the client can decide: Assessment of decision-making capacity*. Minneapolis, MN: University of Minnesota Long-Term Care Decisions Resource Center.

Perspective From Oklahoma

■

Sean Browne

Competency determination is vital in every aspect of case management. In assessment, the client's competency is a determining factor in the validity of the data collected from the client. In developing a care plan, the client's competency will determine the client's ability to participate in the process. A case manager must take into consideration the incompetent client's rights and the client's limited capacity to assume responsibility in implementing and monitoring services.

The case manager's opinion about the client's competence should have some weight with the client and service providers, and even more so in long-standing cases. The case manager has data about the client, family dynamics, and service provider interaction that can be of value in decision making. However, the case manager and those who value her opinion may not have the ultimate power to make the decision. Disagreements are possible, as in the situation of Mrs. R, whose doctor judged her to be incompetent.

There are many ways to resolve such disagreements. In the case of Mrs. R, the physician would normally help develop the care plan as a member of a team or as a consultant to the case manager. The history of physician participation or nonparticipation helps the case manager determine whether a 30-minute consultation could be enough to determine incompetence. In some cases, a second opinion helps resolve disagreements. If there has been an ongoing relationship between the case manager and the client's physician, the need for more formal action might not be necessary. Mrs. R has not been declared incompetent by a court of law. The case manager does not feel Mrs. R is incompetent. Mrs. R seems to have been able to make decisions regarding which of her affairs she is willing to turn over to other family members. Therefore, it appears Mrs. R might be capable of requesting a more thorough evaluation of her own competence which would resolve the disagreement.

To whom is the case manager responsible in assessing the decision-making capabilities of the clients? The clients themselves? Family members? The general public? The case-management program? The answer is probably all of the preceding. Certainly the case manager must be cognizant of the impact of the competency assessment on others, but the case manager's primary responsibility is to the client.

Is it ever ethical to subject incompetent persons to risks to their life and safety? Given our program policy and prevailing community standards, we would answer no. Would it make a difference if the person had made an advance directive? If we were dealing with "living will" issues, perhaps it would make a difference, but living wills do not cover the matters discussed in these cases. Generally there *are* alternatives to putting an incompetent person's life and safety at risk. "Don't ever put me in a nursing home." "I'd rather die than live with my children." "I want to die at home." Case managers must take clients' values into consideration in developing care plans. However, it would not be ethical for a case manager to put such statements ahead of preventing risks to health and safety.

The commentators argue that being locked in a house alone could be a better alternative than a placement away from one's family and familiar milieu. I disagree. In the case of Mrs. S, I wonder about the family's motive for keeping her in her house. Is it a place for the grandson to live? Is it to save nursing home costs, so the inheritance will be larger? Is it to avoid the guilt inherent in "putting mother away"? For whatever reason, this family should be counseled regarding the risks and legal liabilities of locking an incompetent person in a home alone. The laws regarding neglect, and mandatory reporting of this behavior must be considered.

Oklahoma's Eldercare Program, a statewide case-management program based in county health departments, attempts to alleviate ethical dilemmas of this sort in several ways. The case manager tests the client's capacity to participate in the process as early in the relationship as possible. The Mental Status Questionnaire score determines if the client is reliable and when to use an informant in data collection. The completed assessment should reveal any need for further professional evaluation of the client's competence. This program also offers wide flexibility in options that can be presented to the client and family. The case manager's constraints are, of course, service availability and availability of funds. Both of these restrictions could cause the case manager to determine that the case is beyond the scope of the program, and recommend closure and placement of the client in a safer environment.

EDITORS' QUESTIONS FOR FURTHER DISCUSSION

■

1.   Is competency determination special with respect to case management, compared, say, with medical decision-making? Should a case manager's opinion have any weight in an ongoing case

because of the nature and duration of involvement? How should disagreements between case managers and physicians be resolved? How formally should such situations be handled?

2. To whom is the case manager responsible in assessing the decision-making capabilities of the clients? The clients themselves? Family members? The general public? The case-management program?

3. Is it ever ethical to subject incompetent persons to risks to their life and safety? Is a more passive countenancing of unsafe living situations the same as making plans that subject the clients to risk?

4. Would it make a difference if the person had made an advance directive that included these issues?

5. Could it be argued that being locked in a house alone is a better alternative than leaving one's family and familiar surroundings?

6. What practical points might a case manager include in a more detailed assessment of the actual risk to the clients in these cases?

Chapter 6

LIFE-STYLES OF THE NOT-SO-RICH OR FAMOUS: Can Case Managers Serve the Truly Eccentric?

CASE

■

Mrs. A, age 83, lives in a dilapidated shack on the outskirts of town. She has two large dogs that defecate in the house, which is dirty and cluttered. Mrs. A has made a trail in the living room through the debris. Roaches and occasional rodents can be seen scurrying about the house. Because of the filth, the case manager speaks to the client outside in the front yard. Mrs. A has a variety of ailments and should have a regular diet and help with her care. She accepts meals-on-wheels, and the person who delivers the meals says it is a race to see who gets the food first—the client or the roaches.

Mrs. A refuses all other housekeeping or personal care, but how, the case manager wonders, could we send a homemaker or personal care worker there anyway? Always peculiar, she has a few distant relatives who want nothing to do with her. She has not had a physical workup for a long time and avoids doctors.

Mrs. A is not really incompetent. Though she sometimes seems like she's "losing it," when we administer the Mental Status Questionnaire she gets most of the questions right. Based on this screening, she's not incompetent. She says she wants to stay where she is, and she does seem happy with her dogs. If we bring this to a head and get some attention for her, perhaps get her to the hospital for a workup, the dogs will probably be euthanized. What do we do? Close the case? Wait for a crisis? Insist on doing a formal competency workup and hearing? Does it help anyone if she is forced into a nursing home?

The agency gets into situations like this every so often, and they are hard to deal with. Often they involve people who have lived "on the fringe" for most of their lives. Dealing with the cases of alcoholics is particularly difficult. They may not even have a real place to live, and suddenly we get worried about their baths and their meals. Yet, if we leave them alone without adequate medical treatment or hygiene, they probably will die.

The agency has its share of hermit types—people who want to live in the middle of nowhere without electricity. Every year or so, a catman or a catwoman gets referred. At the moment, besides Mrs. A, the agency has Mr. H to worry about. Now in his 80s, he is well known in the community and generally shunned when he comes into town. He never bathes, and, though he doesn't approach people or bother them unless he has a specific question, he is such a sorry sight that children are frightened of him. Though not educated, Mr. H is definitely competent—he even has some instinctive mechanical ability. Until recently, he lived in a shack on his father's land. He has dizzy spells and arthritis that limit his mobility, but he ingeniously has managed to get around in an old electric lawn mower. Recently this conveyance broke down, and he has been unable to get into the nearby larger town to get the necessary part. The case manager has tried to help Mr. H and has arranged for some services including meals that he can pick up at a restaurant in town (they cannot be delivered because the access to his shack is blocked). When Mr. H feels weak and tired now, he lies down on the side of the road and rests. This often happens when he is on the way to pick up his meals. Worried or appalled townspeople have called the 911 emergency number 5 times in the last 3 weeks. Either Mr. H is gone by the time the police and ambulance arrive, or he tells them to go away and let him rest. The public finds this situation unacceptable, as do the police. The case-management agency was put under pressure to take action and have Mr. H's shack condemned. The case manager resisted the pressure, but last week the client's shack mysteriously burned down while the client was off on one of his jaunts. The client was forcibly taken to the hospital and submitted to a bath, and the case manager then found a group home in a different town that reluctantly agreed to admit him on a trial basis. The client hates the care setting, and the other residents wish he was gone too. He's never lived with groups before and doesn't know how to behave. At dinner, he picked up the entire roast pork and took it to his room. He has only been in the group home for 5 days, but he wants to leave and the proprietor wants to eject him.

Mr. H wants to return to his property and rebuild his shack. The program could help by purchasing materials and could even put a used trailer on the property, but the leaders of the community emphatically don't want Mr. H back. They say they will go all the way to the governor about the irresponsibility of the case managers, if that's what it takes. They also say that a sick old man should not be left to die that way.

COMMENTARIES

Case Managers and Eccentric Clients

■

Baruch A. Brody

These two extremely interesting, and unfortunately all too common, cases raise many questions that deserve analysis. This commentary focuses attention on only the following questions: (a) What does competency mean in the setting of case management and how ought it to be determined? (b) What are the obligations of case managers to eccentric but competent clients? (c) What is the role of community sensibilities in the development of an appropriate plan for a client? All three of these questions arise, perhaps in different ways, in both of our cases. I will begin by saying a little about each of these issues in general and then apply the general remarks to the cases at hand.

ANALYSIS OF COMPETENCY

The concept of competency has received extensive discussion in the literature of medical ethics (Buchanan & Brock 1989; Meisel, 1989), and several crucial themes from that literature will be helpful for our setting as well. I would particularly emphasize the themes that competency must always be understood in a task-specific manner, that competency is related to certain capacities, and that competency is a matter of degree. Let us review each of these themes and then apply them to these cases.

Decisional competency must always be understood in a task-specific manner. The question we must always consider is whether a specific individual at a given time is competent to make a specific decision. We must be task-specific because people may be competent to make certain decisions (perhaps because these decisions are less complex or less emotionally charged), while incompetent to make others (which are more complex or emotionally charged). To be sure, some individuals (e.g., the severely demented) may be incompetent to make any decisions, whereas others (e.g., most of us, most of the time) are competent to make all the decisions we face. We must always remember this initial point about competency's being a task-specific notion, because it is precisely those whose competency is questioned who are often competent to make only some decisions.

Task-specific competency is related to possessing certain capacities. Different authors have emphasized different capacities, but I would place primary significance on the ability to receive and remember information, the ability to assess in a reasonable manner the significance of that information, and the ability to reach a decision for which one can give reasons using that information (Brody, 1988). Notice that all of these capacities are process oriented. Competency is not a question of reaching the right decision (even if there is such a thing as the right decision); it is a question of having the capacity to undertake certain decisional processes. We may quite appropriately feel a need to assess competency when unusual decisions are reached, but if the decider gives evidence of the relevant process-oriented capacities, then his or her competency is intact even if the decisions are unusual.

To my mind, but not to the mind of others (Buchanan & Brock, 1989; Meisel, 1989), these first two observations about competency lead to the final observation that competency is best viewed as a matter of degree rather than as an all-or-nothing matter. After all, individuals have these capacities vis-à-vis a given decision to a greater or lesser degree, so it seems reasonable to say that they are competent to make that decision to a greater or lesser degree. This is a more complicated picture than the usual one, for we can no longer say simple (I think, simple-minded) things like we must respect the wishes of the competent but can disregard the wishes of the incompetent. We will need instead to talk in more complex ways about affording greater respect to more competent decisions. But although this approach of degrees of competency is more complex, its complexity rests on the complex truths that the capacities that constitute competency are not possessed in an all-or-nothing manner, and that any attempt to draw a sharp boundary between the competent and incompetent is doomed to arbitrariness and failure.

Let us now apply these three points to Mrs. A and Mr. H. The case descriptions are not as helpful as they might be in light of what we have seen about competency. To begin with, we are not always sure what is the crucial decision in question. In the case of Mrs. A, for example, we're not sure whether the crucial decision is about getting a physical workup for her, or about getting more help in her house, or about placing her in a nursing home. Her competency vis-à-vis each of these decisions may differ, and all of that needs to be distinguished in any analysis of the case. In this respect, the case description of Mr. H. makes it clearer that the crucial decision is about where he is going to live. Second, the assessment of competency in both case descriptions is troubling. Having mechanical ability (what we are told about Mr. H) or passing a Mental Status Questionnaire (what we are told about Mrs. A) is at best very indirect evidence as to whether these individuals possess the relevant capacities for decisional competency vis-à-vis whatever decision we are primarily concerned about when we analyze this case.

Let me present an alternative approach. The first step is to identify the relevant decision with which we are concerned. The second step is to see whether there are reasons for doubting competency. The third step is to identify a process for an initial evaluation of competency by the case manager. The final step is to identify the role, if any, of the courts in this process.

In the case of Mrs. A, there truly are many different questions about which decisions need to be made: Should she have a full physical workup? Should she get more help (e.g., housekeeping) in her current residence? Should she be forced into a nursing home? In the case of Mr. H, the mysterious fire has really left only one major decision, where Mr. H should live. Seeing the different issues (if there are several) in a given case is clearly the first step.

The second step is a crucial threshold step. We normally assume that adults are competent to make decisions for themselves. We should not begin even the most informal assessment of competency unless we have reasons for doubting specific competency. Are they present in this case? The reasons, if there are any, will have to relate to the bizarre quality of the decisions by the clients. We have already suggested that this is acceptable, but we need to be careful not to overextend that point. Mrs. A's decision to stay in her home and her decision to avoid seeing a doctor unless she has a pressing problem are quite common, and it is hard to see how they justify any competency assessment. But her refusal of help with housekeeping and personal care in light of the appalling consequences of that refusal does seem sufficiently bizarre to justify an inquiry into competency. Mr. H's behavior, by way of contrast, seems, in general, sufficiently strange to justify a need to investigate his competency.

How should Mrs. A's competency to make decisions about getting help be assessed? First, she needs to have explained to her what services are available and how they can enable her to maintain herself at home in better conditions, even if they do mean losing some independence. Then, we need to test her to see if she understands and remembers those options and their advantages and disadvantages, and uses that information in reaching a decision. All of this means a lot of discussion with her about her options and her reasons for making whatever decision she makes. To the extent that she shows an inability to remember or understand her options or an inability to use that information in making a decision, we have to that extent reason to doubt her competency. But if she evidences all of that, and decides against help because of the desire to remain as independent as possible, then we must reject our initial suspicion about her competency. In the case of Mr. H., similar discussions must occur, but they will be more complex as they involve the many aspects of choosing a place to reside, so any assessment of the extent of his competency vis-à-vis the relevant decision is going to be more complex.

Notice that nothing has been said so far about any role for the legal system. That is not an omission. I believe that the legal system has no role before an assessment by a clinician or a case manager provides serious reasons, in light of an assessment of capacities, for doubting competency vis-à-vis the relevant decision. Then, and only then, should a formal petition be made to a court, in part to provide a formal review in an adversarial setting in which the client can challenge the assessment and in part to provide the formal authorization required for coercive intervention. Turning to the courts before then seems to be rushing things without justification by unfairly challenging the client's competency without an adequate preliminary investigation.

OBLIGATIONS TO ECCENTRIC CLIENTS

Eccentric clients, like noncompliant patients, challenge providers in many ways. In this section, I discuss a set of obligations that case managers have toward these clients, about the limits of those obligations, and about their practical implications.

The first, and most fundamental, of these obligations is to respect clients, even if they are eccentric. This notion of respect must not be misunderstood. Mr. H's behavior in the group home or Mrs. A's willingness to live in appalling filth may be deserving of no respect. We may well be justified in saying that they are poor decisions, representing pathological failures of adequate social and personal development. This first obligation only calls on us to respect these individuals (in ways that will be discussed later), not necessarily their decisions. All too often, professionals walk away from these individuals, taking their eccentric decisions as personal repudiations, rather than as expression of other values, and this tendency must be avoided.

The second obligation is to give these clients a fair assessment of their competency. The more they are competent, the more we must abide by their decisions. When we see those decisions as ill founded, we are tempted to just say that those who make them are incompetent. Part of fulfilling the obligation to respect the client, even if one does not respect the decision, is to follow the previously outlined process for ascertaining competency so as to ensure that the client's decision is not inappropriately disregarded. The significance of this point cannot be overstated. Especially when there is significant community pressure, as in the case of Mr. H, it is all so easy to manipulate the system to get a formal determination of the eccentric client's incompetency, regardless of the truth. Resorting to that technique is, to my mind, a paradigm case of failing to respect individuals. What can be less respectful than denying a person's decisional authority over themselves when they actually have decisional competency?

The third obligation is to be imaginative, an obligation that is present in different forms depending on what degree of competency is ascribed to the client. This obligation is usually not mentioned, so I want to say a lot more about it because I feel it is very crucial.

Suppose that it is decided that Mrs. A is sufficiently competent about making the decision to get extra help so that her refusal of that help should not be overridden. Some would say that the case manager is relieved of any further responsibility until a crisis arises. Some would say that the case manager has at most the obligation to periodically reoffer the help to Mrs. A. I find that second approach better, because the first approach, to my mind, comes close to taking the refusal as personal and therefore walking away from the case. But I find that second account inadequate, precisely because it seems so unimaginative. Those who are proud of their independence find it difficult to take help even when it is offered, and a mere repetition of the offer is not likely to get very far. Imaginative offers may do much better, and that is why I talk about the obligation to be imaginative. It is hard to discuss the precise nature of an imaginative offer in the case of Mrs. A because one needs to know a lot more both about her and about her problems to design such an offer. But in the case of Mr. H, it seems easier to indicate at least one example. Mr. H's being in a sudden crisis was related to his lying down on the side of the road when he went to town to get the arranged meals. Nothing more imaginative than having the meals delivered or helping him to fix the old lawn mower so that he could ride to town to get his meals might have avoided the sudden crisis. The former is hardly imaginative (it is what Mrs. A is getting). The latter is a bit unusual, but it would give him more general mobility. Good case managers are obliged to be imaginative vis-à-vis their sufficiently competent patients, and they need to have the authority to do imaginative things, if they are to be able to provide needed services without coercing sufficiently competent clients.

There is an important institutional issue that needs to be raised here about the extent to which case managers ought to have the liberty to design a package of services, even if they are very nonstandard, which meet the needs of the client. What restrictions, if any, on the type of services that can be provided are justified? How much authority to design nonstandard packages should be given to case managers and how much to their clients? These cases remind us that there is a need to confront these institutional issues, even if this case commentary is not the place to do so.

This same point about being imaginative, with somewhat different emphases, needs to be made about the obligations of case managers to clients like Mrs. A and Mr. H when they are judged to be sufficiently incompetent vis-à-vis a specific decision so that coercive interventions are justified. Interventions that are coercive (e.g., you will not be able to live where you want to live and must go to a different setting) can be performed in many ways, and imagination can often provide a way that is far more acceptable to the clients, even if it is not what they really want. Here, the notion of degrees of competency and incompetency is very important. The more incompetent the client is, the less reason there is to attend to their wishes. But the more capacities they continue to have, even if they are not adequate to justify decisional independence, the more we are obligated to search out imaginative compromises that are at least partially responsive to their wishes.

An important comment about the limitations on this obligation to be imaginative is needed at this point. Being imaginative often requires time, resources, and institutional flexibility. When they are in short supply, it may literally become impossible to be imaginative in the ways required. Even when possible, case mangers must allocate time and resources among all of their clients, and this inevitably means that not all imaginative possibilities can be explored and implemented. Accepting all of these implications of a world of limited resources only means accepting limitations on the obligation to be imaginative. It should not be used as an excuse to reject the obligation.

One final observation. It is commonplace to talk of the obligation to serve as an advocate for clients. I find that way of talking acceptable but insufficient. Being imaginative is a way of being an advocate, and I like the language of imagination because it stresses a mode of effective advocacy.

COMMUNITY SENSIBILITIES

For a long time, the liberal tradition (and I use that term in the broadest sense) has emphasized that individuals ought to be free to do what they want to do so long as it doesn't harm others. Others may be offended by your behavior, but as long as you do not harm them, they cannot interfere coercively to stop you from exercising that freedom. Of course, this rule applies only to competent adult individuals, and that is why we wind up spending so much time assessing competency.

This liberal tradition has in particular emphasized the need of the community to accept what may be offensive to most individuals as long as those engaging in the behavior do not harm other individuals. Thus, for example, liberals have fought for the right of consenting adults to view pornography, to engage in a variety of sexual practices, and so on. Even in this tradition, however, exceptions are made when offensive behavior becomes public and then directly intrudes on others. In his recent restatement of the liberal tradition, Joel Feinberg has emphasized the right of society to stop sufficiently public offensive behavior. Of course, all of these discussions have primarily focused on the criminal law (e.g., should pornography be legal), but they can be applied to our cases. Let us discuss the issue of the legitimacy of considering the public offensiveness of client behavior in making decisions about their case management.

This issue is less significant in the case of Mrs. A. She lives on the outskirts of town, and nothing is said in the case description about her offending others. No doubt, many members of the community would be offended or disgusted by how she lives, but she doesn't intrude into their lives. As Feinberg (1985) has pointed out, offense or disgust in cases of mere knowledge of the offensive or disgusting behavior constitutes a weak case for intervention.

The issue is much more significant in the case of Mr. H. Others are appalled by his lying on the side of the road and find it unacceptable that he just lie there. They don't want him and his problems intruding on them in the public arena. In thisrespect, Mr. H is like so many of the homeless that many urban residents are forced to encounter on a daily basis.

Two observations are in place. The first is to draw a contrast between the members of Mr. H's community and the urban citizens who want the homeless out of the way. The members of Mr. H's community don't just want him out of sight. They want the agency to provide for him a place to live. This is, alas, often not the case in the contemporary urban setting. Second, and this is a point that Feinberg emphasizes, the extent of the community's legitimate right to avoid being offended in the public arena is dependent on the extent of the actual offense to reasonable people. Mr. H's lying there by the side of the road may trouble people (who wonder why he isn't being helped), but being troubled is not the same thing as being offended. Legitimate community interests should be considered in an appropriate way, but we need to be careful not to overstate those interests. The members of the community who probably have the greatest claim against Mr. H's offensive behavior are the other residents in the care facility who quite understandably want him out.

Many will find these last remarks troubling. Aren't we required by the principle of respect for persons to put up with a lot of unusual and even offensive behavior on the part of eccentric individuals? We certainly are, but we are not required to put up with everything. The more the behavior is offensive, and the more we cannot avoid it because it is present in public space or it intrudes on our private space, the more we have a legitimate demand to be considered in planning with and for eccentric individuals.

CONCLUSION

There is not enough information provided in the case description to answer the questions that need to be answered. I have, instead, provided a framework for case managers who confront cases like these two cases.

REFERENCES

Buchanan, A. E. and Brock, D. (1989) *Deciding for others*. New York: Cambridge University Press.

Brody, B. A. (1988). *Life and death decision making* (pp.100-104). New York: Oxford University Press.

Feinberg, J. (1985). *Offense to others.* New York: Oxford University Press.

Meisel, A. (1989). *The right to die.* New York: Wiley.

The Burden of Beneficence

■

Bart J. Collopy

Mrs. A and Mr. H test the very limits of what it means to be a *client.* Both of them are fierce loners who have chosen to stay as much as possible beyond the reach ("the clutches," they would undoubtedly say) of organized beneficence. But advancing age and frailty make their self-dependence increasingly risky and draw them inevitably, even if involuntarily, into the orbits of "cliency." Despite their idiosyncracies, then, Mrs. A and Mr. H raise questions relevant to any one of us in our aging, questions about self-determination and dependency, the obligations and powers of care providers, the amount of tolerance or control we will find when we become frail and want, still, to go our own ways.

In pursuing these questions I focus on beneficence, that commitment to the well-being of clients that can so powerfully dominate cases involving the frail elderly. In particular I explore the ways in which beneficence can be intrusive; the nature of "long-term" as opposed to "acute episode" beneficence; the use of beneficence as a cover for community control; and, finally, the tasks of social mediation that beneficence creates for case managers and their agencies.

INTRUSIVE BENEFICENCE

Clearly, the case management agency feels strong pressures to intervene more forcefully and improve the lot of Mrs. A and Mr. H. Beneficence of this sort is a fundamental professional value, not lightly set aside. Indeed, it would be psychologically difficult and morally questionable for case managers to void their commitment to a client's well-being at the first glimpse of an autonomous refusal. Standards of care are bred into the bones of conscientious providers, however meagerly they may count with clients themselves. Thus, it obviously cuts against the professional and moral grain of providers to have a frail client, like Mrs. A, living in filth and poverty, without adequate nutrition or health care. Beneficence urges case managers to get a complete medical workup for her and a competency hearing; it nettles them with doubts about simply leaving her alone until a more serious crisis develops.

But Mrs. A wants to be left alone. "She has always been peculiar," we are told. She is happy with her dogs, accustomed, it seems, to the dirt and clutter of the shack that the case manager finds impassable. Moreover the shack is *home* to her, a place to be protected, perhaps fortressed, against the help she considers invasive.

Forcing more care on Mrs. A would clearly deny her autonomy in the name of her well-being *as defined by others*. True, her inattention to medical care may be imprudent, but it is the kind of risk that adults are generally allowed to take without facing the risk of involuntary hospitalization. The prospect that forced hospitalization might be coupled with the euthanasia of her dogs gives a cruel twist to a beneficent intervention. And it is hard to see what this hospitalization would accomplish in the long run, if Mrs. A were free to return to her (now dogless) shack and her usual shunning of doctors. Of course, hospitalization might be a first step toward involuntary placement in a nursing home, a transfer that could be authorized by a court-appointed guardian after a competency hearing. But a competency hearing would subject Mrs. A to a process that is mired in confused and conflicting definitions of competency, in stereotypes about mental decline among the elderly, and in medical-legal biases against risk taking (Coleman & Dooley, 1990; Iris, 1988, 1990). Moreover, the case manager finds Mrs. A sufficiently competent, despite her occasional lapses.

The issue of competency, or decisional capacity, is of course a crucial one, because lack of capacity is a primary justification for overruling the choices and controlling the behavior of the frail elderly. Clients who are eccentric *and* elderly face double jeopardy in this regard. Their social aberrations can be considered mental aberrations; their physical frailty taken as sign of cognitive frailty; their occasional lapses seen as proof of lasting incapacity (Katz, 1984; McCullough, 1984). Such judgments have powerful force in the absence of more thorough clinical and moral assessments (President's Commission, 1982; Tancredi, 1987). But case managers should be uneasy with solutions that cut through knotted cases with a single morally relieving stroke. Problematic cases can be too easily solved by an assessment of "incapacity" for case managers to adopt anything but high caution in this area. When a client is characterized as eccentric and, like Mrs. A, lives beyond the latitudes of standard behavior, there is real risk that she will lose the standard protections accorded autonomy.

It is crucial, then, that eccentricity not be identified with mental illness or incapacity. The dangers of labeling are very real here. Thomas Szasz (1961) may overstate the case when he argues that "mental illness" is simply a medical label for socially aberrant behavior. But he rightly alerts us to the kind of category mistake that sees eccentricity as mental illness—and eccentrics, therefore, as individuals to be cared for under force. Although Mrs. A is certainly eccentric, her refusal of additional care appears quite authentic, because it echoes her past moral history and character. From her lifelong perspective she is acting coherently and reasonably. Forcing care on her would be an indefensible breach of her autonomy, dignity, past life, and—strange as it may seem to some—her present happiness.

"LONG HAUL" BENEFICENCE

Although respect for Mrs. A's autonomy, dignity, and happiness argues against forced care or coercion to change her life-style, it does not ease the burden of beneficence—the basic commitment of case managers to the well-being of their clients. Mrs. A's case manager could immediately pull back in the name of Mrs. A's autonomous right to deteriorate, alone, in her dog-messed shack, although such disconnection would suggest a model of care in which providers simply "service" clients' autonomous choices. In this model, the promptings of beneficence would be obediently quieted by the autonomy of clients—an autonomy most powerfully felt in the *negative* right to be left alone.

A more complex model of care would admit (even *require*) the moral pain case managers experience in the face of some client choices. This deep troubling of case managers would stem from their beneficent concern for their clients' well-being and from their commitment to their clients' *positive* rights—rights to enhanced living, larger options, and long-term as well as immediate autonomy. In the case of Mrs. A, then, the case management agency would find itself in real moral tension— trying to respect her autonomy and trying not to abandon her to choices that bode badly for her future well-being and autonomy. In short, the agency has the hard task of continuing to be concerned for Mrs. A's welfare even though she clearly pulls back from this concern.

There may be clients who so adamantly refuse assistance that agencies finally have no recourse but to close the case. But this is an extreme response, and beneficence requires that it be reached reluctantly, only after strenuous efforts to find some mutually acceptable and workable plan of care. In practice, those managing and providing community-based service usually go to great lengths to continue service and contact with elderly clients even in the face of noncompliance and refusal of care. The operative model of care is not a narrowly "contractual" one that requires a client to accept a proffered care plan or else be rejected by the agency.

If the principle of autonomy precludes forcing services on Mrs. A, the principle of beneficence precludes abandoning her when she chooses to reject most of the care offered. She may have accepted only minimal assistance, but she *has* established some relationship with the case-management agency, and this relationship, prickly as it may be, ought to be sustained. Furthermore, this is a long-term care situation. Mrs. A has refused housekeeping services, not dialysis or tube feeding. There may be time, then, to navigate the shoals of her refusal. Her decision, like many in long-term care, does not exhibit the terribly short linkage between refusal and result that marks acute care decisions—especially the paradigm termination-of-treatment decisions. Long-term care has the advantage (and burden) of time, of ongoing contact, the long haul of a case. This means that care providers often have room for maneuvering, for inching toward mutual understanding and trust, trying the paths of accommodation, negotiation, incremental coaxing, partial solutions, time trials—all the various strategies that can respect autonomy and yet further beneficence (Agich, 1990; Collopy, Dubler, Zuckerman, 1990; Moody, 1988).

Conversely, attempts to bring fuller care to resisting clients do not always succeed, and if Mrs. A's case-management agency makes no progress, it may have to fall back on a waiting strategy. The agency could stay with her case on limited terms, keeping in contact when possible, waiting for some opportunity to increase care without forcing it on her. This is not an easy path for care providers to take. The "opportunity" for more care may come only with further deterioration in Mrs. A's health or mental capacity or living conditions. Case managers know, up close, the burdens of watching a client's decline. They are not likely to romanticize eccentricity or underestimate its costs in the midst of old age and frailty. A waiting strategy is liable to be felt, then, not as a splendid defense of the principle of autonomy so much as a troubling, morally ambiguous choice prompted by beneficence.

Questions can be raised here about the resources available to case managers as they struggle with such hard choices. By and large, home care and other service agencies do not have access to the resources that have been developed in acute care to assist physicians and nurses facing ethical dilemmas. In long-term care in general and community-based services in particular, there has been little *systematic* discussion of ethical issues. Professionals and agencies have certainly struggled with these issues but in a "privatized" fashion—as isolated individuals or agencies facing ethical problems as they arise in their practice. They have not had access to the ethics resources available in acute care: institutional ethics committees, ethics education programs on the preservice and in-service levels, ethics consults or "grand rounds," the discussion of ethical issues in professional publications and conferences, the development of case studies, commentaries, and wider research focusing on the ethics of community-based programs.

From its side, bioethics has been so fixated on acute care issues that it has done little to develop familiarity with, much less resources for, long-term care providers. In short, the limited discussion of ethical quandaries routinely faced by case managers emphasizes the barely germinal state of long-term care ethics.

BENEFICENCE AND COMMUNITY CONTROL

The case of Mr. H replicates many of the issues already raised in the case of Mrs. A. Again, a frail but mentally capable client follows a difficult and idiosyncratic path, accepting only very limited assistance. But Mr. H introduces an additional ethical tangle. He is troublesome to the local community. He comes into town, unbathed and unkempt, frightening children, lying down on the side of the road to rest, dismissing the emergency teams who rush to his aid. When his shack suddenly burns down, the opportunity to institutionalize him is seized. He is forcibly hospitalized, "submitted" to a bath, and relocated to a group home in a different town. In the eyes of some, his lot has been improved; the town, certainly, has been relieved of a problematic presence.

But Mr. H hates the home. And his relocation turns out to be a quickly fraying solution. In dramatic proof that idiosyncratic clients are not "standardized" by group settings, Mr. H walks off with the whole roast at dinner. He continues to chart his own strange course, now inflicting his eccentricity in concentrate on a small enclosed group rather than on the larger community. After 5 days, the other residents and the home's management want him ejected.

And Mr. H himself is desperate to get out. He wants to return to the family property where he has always lived, wants to rebuild his ruined shack. The case-management agency could facilitate this return, but the "leaders of the community" stand against such efforts. They do not want "a sick old man . . . left alone to die" in a shack. Their opposition is framed beneficently, but it is nonetheless coercive and controlling. Mr. H is a mentally competent, authentic loner who wants to go on living as he always has. In short, he seems quite willing to die on the terms he has lived. The shack is his home, the family property his place, eremitical life his mode. There is little indication that, back at his old homesite, he would describe himself as a sick old man left alone to die.

Of course, beneficence might not be the only force at work in the decision to institutionalize Mr. H. The community leaders may not want this unkempt, troublesome old man wandering their streets any longer. The danger for the case-management agency is that, under the rubric of beneficence, it may be used as an instrument of community control. The agency might decide against resettling Mr. H in his former place if the resources required were massive or if helping him meant denying equally crucial assistance to others. But this does not seem to be the case. In fact, caring for Mr. H in a group home could be more expensive in the long run. His recent behavior forecasts large troubleshooting tasks for the agency, perhaps constant efforts to find new placements as he makes off with more dinner roasts.

In the end, the agency's moral imperatives favor advocacy for Mr. H's autonomy rather than the "social gatekeeping" role that the community leaders want. Put more bluntly, the agency should not take on behavior control tasks at the community's bidding. An agency ought to be extremely reluctant to institutionalize elderly individuals because the community finds them indecorous or otherwise troublesome. Enforcing community standards in this fashion turns "clients" into "charges" and vacates the agency's advocacy role, its commitment to clients' autonomy and their *self-defined* well-being. In the present case, then, the agency would be right to refuse cooperation. If the community wants to move eccentric elderly out of its midst, it can take this on directly and not press the case-management agency to do its patrolling. Let the community leaders "go all the way to the governor," if they want.

Easy for an outsider to suggest? Quite true. The fiscal and political risks of being confrontational with community leaders could work against the agency's service to other clients. A more tempered solution would suggest a mediating and educating role for the agency, a response that is ironic rather than confrontational. Conversely, this mediating role is no small task, something of a puzzle even.

MEDIATING TASKS OF BENEFICENCE

Case-management agencies do more than serve clients in the community. In effect, they actually embody the community's response—or lack of response-to its dependent elderly and young, its poor, homeless, and otherwise needy members. To the extent that community agencies are the moral proving grounds of public policy and social responsibility, they help a community face and fathom the human misery in its midst. Agencies do not simply "take care" of these problems by removing them from public view, though we might wish they did.

In addition to serving their clients, then, agencies have a "penumbral" mission to the wider community, a mission that becomes critical when clients and communities clash. In the case of Mr. H, the agency faces the difficult task of shaping the community's sensibility about the dependent elderly, their potential eccentricities, and the inevitable burdens that a growing elderly population entails for the community. And Mr. H *is* a burden. A defense of his eccentric life-style can be easily mounted from the ethics of autonomy, but responding to his odorous presence or his naps on the street, or trying to deal with his asocial behavior in a group home, can honestly test the tolerance of both care providers and the wider community.

The task of mediating between clients and community is, in essence, a task of translating the autonomy and dignity of someone like Mr. H from abstract principle to fleshy presence. There are few immediate clues about how this might be done. Bioethics has much to say about *getting to* decisions that respect autonomy, but it provides little treatment of the moral tasks that follow *in the wake* of such decisions. Surely one of these tasks is to mediate between an individual like Mr. H and the community that chokes on his autonomous behavior, even if it tolerates it. But how can an unsympathetic community come to see the value of the eccentric's autonomy, come perhaps to recognize the common human bone under the seemingly strange skin? Where are the moral guides for *this* task?

Mulling over Mrs. A and her dogs and Mr. H, the sorry sight who frightens children, I thought of Dylan Thomas's "The Hunchback in the Park" (1957). Thomas is neither case manager nor ethicist, but perhaps he offers some moral support to those who provide services to the eccentric, to clients who are strangely and "inappropriately" autonomous. Thomas's poem describes a hunchback who inhabits the local park all day, eating bread from a newspaper, drinking water from the chained cup that the children fill with gravel, taunted by the boys of the town who run in hunchbacked mockery from his anger, sleeping at night, unchained, in a dog kennel.

Out of this eccentric life the old man summons up a shape not strange at all, but primal and communal. In the park, alone, among the nurses and the swans, the old dog sleeper

Made all day until bell time
A woman figure without fault
Straight as a young elm

Straight and tall from his crooked bones
That she might stand in the night
After the locks and chains

All night in the unmade park
After the railings and shrubberies
The birds the grass the trees the lake
And the wild boys innocent as strawberries
Had followed the hunchback
To his kennel in the dark.

REFERENCES

Agich, G. J. (1990). Reassessing autonomy in long term care. *Hastings Center Report, 20,* 12–17.

Coleman, N., & Dooley, J. (1990). Making the guardianship system work. *Generations, 14* (Suppl.), 47–50.

Collopy, B. J., Dubler, N. N., & Zuckerman, C. (1990). The ethics of home care: Autonomy and accommodation. *Hastings Center Report, 20* (Special Suppl.), 1–16.

Iris, M. A. (1988). Guardianship and the elderly: A multi-perspective view of the decisionmaking process. *The Gerontologist, 28* (Suppl.), 39–45.

Iris, M. A. (1990). Threats to autonomy in guardianship decision making. *Generations, 14* (Suppl.), 39–41.

Katz, J. (1984). *The silent world of doctor and patient.* New York: Free Press.

McCullough, L. B. (1984). Medical care for elderly patients with diminished competence: An ethical analysis. *Journal of the American Geriatrics Society, 32,* 150–153.

Moody, H. R. (1988). From informed consent to negotiated consent. *The Gerontologist, 28* (Suppl.), 64–70.

Presidents Commission for the Study of Ethical Problems in Medicine and Biomedical and Behavioral Research. (1982). *Making health care decisions.* Washington, DC: Government Printing Office.

Szasz, T. S. (1961). *The myth of mental illness.* New York: Harper & Row.

Tancredi, L. R. (1987). The mental status examination. *Generations, 11,* 24–31.

Thomas, D. (1957). *The collected poems of Dylan Thomas.* New York: New Directions.

Tensions Between Person and Community

■

Stephen G. Post

She would not exchange her solitude for anything. Never again to be forced to move to the rhythms of others. For in this solitude she had won to a reconciled peace. . . . Now he was violating it with his constant campaigning: Sell the house and move to the Haven. (You sit, you sit—there too you could sit like a stone.)
—Tillie Olsen, *Tell Me a Riddle*

It is not unusual for competent or marginally competent elderly people to cling to residential roots, because this assures a sense of continuity with their biographical pasts. This theme is the focus of my commentary. Immediately, however, it must be noted that elderly people with degrees of memory loss can sometimes carry out activities of daily living in their old familiar environs, but fail in these activities when moved to a new residence because they can no longer learn the map of novel surroundings. Putting this functional aspect of relocation aside, I will concentrate on the notions of existential meaning and rootedness in places of personal memory.

As Spar and LaRue write, "The search for continuity may be at the heart of reminiscence, which occurs at all ages, and of the process of life review that is so common among elderly adults" (1990, p. 21). Ruptures with the past through events such as forced relocation can violate the search for continuity and result in considerable anomie. In one case with which I am familiar, a 75-year-old man with increasingly severe dementia resisted relocation to a group home. He lived on the shores of Lake Erie in a small shack, overlooking the waves where his father had died in a sudden storm while sailing, and where the ashes of his prematurely deceased eldest son had been sprinkled some years ago. From Greek myths to Tillie Olsen's classic *Tell Me a Riddle*, growing old has meaning as a journey home, to this specific land with these particular layers of meaning (Bagnell & Soper, 1989; Yahnke & Eastman, 1990).

To understand the moral significance of place in the lives of many elderly people requires more than a theoretical appeal to respect for autonomy. It requires appreciation of the psychological harm inflicted on elderly people when they are coercively removed from places of meaning. What is to the external observer nothing but a beat up old shack at the outskirts of town may represent all of the memories and associations that made the life of an old man or woman worth living. To strip elderly people of their meaningful places is a severe step that may result in a tragic downward spiral of depression and failure to thrive. Our society is already one of anomie, or as Peter Berger describes it, of "the homeless mind." The individual's sense of community and belonging may be deeply dependent on an old environment, with its power to bring to mind life events and rites of passage.

Claims that relocation is in the best interests of the client who resists it may in some cases be valid. Prospectively it can be very difficult for the case manager to predict the final outcome of relocation, positive or negative, with respect to the psychological and related physical well-being of the client. Ethically, we refer here to the notion of moral "probabilism." This term was developed by the 17th-century "casuists" (from the Latin for "case") as they worked through particular moral cases on the assumption that ethics is often an *inexact* art admitting only degrees of certainty, as Aristotle insisted. What the case manager needs is what some contemporary philosophers term "moral luck." Regarding relocation and elderly people, there is a gray zone in which the case manager will not be sure of the rightness of a decision until it can be retrospectively assessed, as is the case with almost all practical reasoning.

Respect for place, for the very crucible of life meaning in the case of some elderly people, is part of what any sensitive commitment to the client's good must include. Here respect for client autonomy is coincidental or coextensive with beneficence, that is, with the client's good. Respect for place is crucial to the client's sense of self-esteem and identity. If client preferences are overridden unnecessarily, whatever good might have been intended will be threatened. There are, of course, cases in which respect for autonomy leaves an elderly person in such severe risk and peril that a strong paternalistic intervention is justified. Unfortunately, for the case manager, there are no ethical theories that will solve these dilemmas a priori; any moral success will emerge from the reasoning of experienced case managers, guided by an appreciation of autonomy and beneficence as midlevel principles that can be coextensive or conflictual depending on the particulars of any given case. Now on to two cases, Mr. H and Mrs. A, "probabilistically" considered.

MR. H

Mr. H was living in a shack on his father's land. He presumably feels emotionally tied to that land, though we do not have the thick case description that might verify this presumption. So long as Mr. H is competent, he should be permitted to live on this land, despite the community's intolerance of his eccentricity.

His old electric lawn mower should be fixed. Apparently, this would require nothing more than securing for him the necessary mechanical part. Had this been accomplished, Mr. H would never have had to take the walks into town that left him resting by the road, an eyesore to the community. The case manager could easily have solved Mr. H's problems, at least for the short term, by correcting a small mechanical difficultly.

I am reminded of a case in Cleveland in which social workers were inclined to remove a slightly demented woman from her apartment because of stifling heat. The elder health care team decided, as a reasonable alternative, to send in a carpenter to free up the windows that had been painted shut. The woman is still residing happily in her home.

In the case of Mr. H., his shack burned down—one suspects arson—and he was forcibly taken to a hospital, eventually to a group home. After several days of group living, he wants to return to his land and rebuild the shack. The case manager could provide him with some building materials (he is skilled with his hands) and a used trailer. There is no reason not to do so.

As in many such cases, the community puts pressure on the case manager. The leaders of the community do not want Mr. H back. At this point, only one essential question needs to be asked: Are not moral values more important than aesthetic ones? The good of Mr. H appears tied to respecting his desire to return home. He is clearly not thriving in a new and unwanted environment. All the necessary resources are available to implement his wishes. One can be suspicious of the community's statements of concern about the welfare of Mr. H. Whatever moral idealism the community may express could easily be little more than a thin veneer over an evidently seething cauldron of aesthetically based intolerance. Let the community take the case all the way to the governor, but protect Mr. H with the full weight of law.

This sort of tension between community and the rights of elderly people is hardly uncommon. It occurs regularly in disposition planning from geriatric clinics and elder health centers. In a recent case, an elderly poet who founded the Cleveland Poetry Society had not bathed properly for several years, nor had she painted her home. The neighborhood association, with the help of local authorities, was able to have her brought into University Hospitals for a competency evaluation. She looked filthy, with dirt and feces packed thickly under her uncut fingernails. She described herself to a department psychiatrist as a neopagan white wicca (witch) feminist no longer conforming to the ways of her neighbors. The psychiatrist, despite powerful denunciation from the community, judged her competent. She returned to her home, and members of the society began to mow her lawn monthly. In this case, the psychiatrist stood on high moral ground.

MRS. A

As for the case of Mrs. A, age 83, living on the outskirts of town in a dilapidated shack, again ethics must take precedence over aesthetics. Mrs. A is at liberty to live in a dirty and cluttered house. Perhaps the case manager might negotiate with Mrs. A to have roach and rodent control implemented, albeit such creatures are remarkably resilient. Mrs. A needs a regular diet, and she does fortunately accept meals-on-wheels. Evidently she is willing to take mental status tests, which she passes.

In the case of Mrs. A, it is difficult to surmise why she wishes to remain in her shack. Nothing indicates that the place itself has special meaning for her, although we need to know more about this. She does love her two dogs, despite their defecating in the house. The dogs have apparently not been house trained. Perhaps Mrs. A would consent to some advice from a dog trainer on this matter. Given the importance of her relationship with the dogs, the case manager should assure Mrs. A that should she agree to a hospital workup, the dogs would be taken care of, rather than euthanized. Maybe, if Mrs. A knew that her dogs would be well cared for by others, she would gradually consider moving to a nursing home, especially if she could bring a picture of her dogs with her. As Waymack and Taler have written, "remembrances from the home should be brought to the new location" (1988, p. 204). We need to know more about Mrs. A's reasons for wanting to live on the outskirts of town, so that possible psychological harms can be avoided. Understanding and negotiation are called for. What makes her life meaningful, and how can these meanings be respected?

It would be helpful to ask Mrs. A why she shuns doctors. She may have had an unpleasant relationship with a physician in the past, and adheres to some negative stereotypes of doctors from which she could be dissuaded. Possibly Mrs. A was abused by her presumably deceased husband and will only express her thoughts to a woman case manager (Grau, 1989). The case manager should make every effort to clear up any misunderstandings or other obstacles that might prevent Mrs. A from freely pursuing necessary medical interventions. However, if Mrs. A's wishes are in fact not based on misunderstandings and related fears, then the case manager will have to await a crisis before intervening.

GENERAL QUESTIONS RAISED

These cases raise a number of general questions. First, is the distinction between eccentricity and mental illness possible or relevant for case managers? Certainly the case manager should have a comprehensive understanding of the wide array of commonly encountered emotional disorders among elderly people. Dementia, depression, suspiciousness, agitation, anxiety, sleeping disorders, and bereavement are all phenomena with which the case manager should be broadly familiar (Blazer, 1990). However, unless these difficulties are severe and seriously threaten the welfare of a client, draconian measures should be avoided. Eccentricity, after all, is a form of nonconformism that deserves tolerance. If Mr. H wants to ride an old electric lawn mower, that is his business. Case managers should avoid the "tyranny of the normal."

Under what circumstances should a case manager encourage a formal competency determination? There is no need for routine testing of competency with elderly people merely because they are old. If, in the course of conversation, a client appears unable to understand his or her situation, fails to understand disclosed information, and is unable to "give risk/benefit-related reasons" (Beauchamp and Childress, 1989, p. 85), then a competency test is necessary. However, in the gray zone of marginal competence, where a client's competency is difficult to measure, a case manager should be reluctant to err on the side of safety. Mrs. A is "not really incompetent," but because she sometimes sounds as if she is "losing it," superficial testing is justified. Because Mrs. A passed the Mental Status Questionnaire quite easily, it would be wrong to take coercive actions for a formal competency workup and hearing. Had she done poorly on the test, then a strong argument could be made for such actions. The case manager should retest Mrs. A periodically. Mr. H, however, is "definitely competent." There is no evidence to the contrary. Therefore, a competency test is uncalled for.

Case managers should not use competency tests loosely, or as a means to prematurely strip the client of autonomy. Conversely, incompetent clients need protections. Often, a client will be competent with respect to some activities, but not others. On the continuum of partial competency, a client's values and wishes should be respected as much as possible. Whatever areas of experience are within the client's range of competency should be preserved from coercion.

How should community sensibilities or community outrage influence the case-management program? Here I am committed to the good of the client, inclusive of the psychological benefits of control over location. There has never been a time when eccentricity has not been denounced as a threat to the community; nor has there been a time when communities have fully avoided scapegoating people who are different. I suggest a somewhat amused response to nonconformity, a bit of the humorous. Foucault points out that before the Enlightenment, Western culture was much more tolerant of seemingly irrational behaviors. Only with the 17th century did communities no longer find unreason of "instructive value" (1965, p. 78). Granted, communities must protect their incompetent members from harm. So also they must avoid scapegoating those who are different.

Indeed, I would argue that Mr. H makes a very important contribution to his community—his presence helps people to accept diversity and difference. The community is enriched by being faithful to his presence and should pitch in to build the shack, with Mr. H's permission. With our societal inclination to rigid standards of beauty, physical prowess, and productivity, it is easy to wrongly assume that people who are different must therefore be suffering. Leslie A. Fiedler has written of a "deep ambivalence toward fellow creatures who are perceived at any given moment as disturbingly deviant, outside currently acceptable physiological norms" (1985, p. 152). He refers to "a vestigial primitive fear of the abnormal." "Perhaps," he writes, "it is especially important for us to realize that finally there are no normals, at a moment when we are striving desperately to eliminate freaks, to normalize the world" (1985, p. 157). The novelist Dostoyevsky made great use of idiot epileptic figures as salvific for community (1955).

To what extent should the case manager determine the risks clients can incur? If a case manager finds that a client's environment is especially risky, then a stronger argument can be made for relocation based on marginal competency. However, relocation should be a last resort after efforts to mitigate risk through reasonable environmental modifications. The manager's ideal is to support client preferences through risk minimization. Yet risk can never be eliminated from the human environment, and people must accept this, as the nursing home ombudsman will insist. It is wrong to eliminate human freedom in the conceptually flawed endeavor to eliminate risk fully.

Once a case manager is involved, is he or she obligated to try to correct substandard living conditions? I believe so. In the case of both Mrs. A and Mr. H, there were opportunities to improve living conditions in their shacks. An exterminator could be called to get rid of roaches, and a small mechanical part might easily have been delivered to Mr. H. If a trailer is available for Mr. H, then it should be secured. This is the sort of modest ingenuity that preserves meaning and makes the lives of clients worth living.

TELL ME A RIDDLE

As a final comment, it is important to consider the question of relocation as a gender issue. Elderly men are most likely to be cared for in their homes by their wives, who generally outlive them. Given the life-span differences between men and women in our culture, it is more probable that case managers will be dealing with women as relocation decisions are forged. It might be quite helpful for case managers to be exposed to some of the literature in the field of women's studies regarding the matter of relocation. Women who have relocated frequently, sometimes following a husband's career moves, can struggle repeatedly with the loss of community and the necessity of making new friendships. Or they may not have moved frequently, but are at a stage of life where solitude is highly valued as a respite from decades of child rearing.

While a humanities professor at a women's college, I taught a considerable number of older women students, and I discovered that relocation is a feminist issue. Without question, the best articulation of this issue comes from Tillie Olsen, with her novella *Tell Me a Riddle*, winner of the O'Henry Award. It describes in powerful terms the anguish a woman can feel when threatened with relocation toward the end of her life, when she has finally been able to achieve a degree of solitude and independence from familial tasks. The study of Olsen's brief work can raise consciousness, and perhaps mitigate unnecessary coercive interventions.

REFERENCES

Bagnell, P., & Soper, P. S. (1989). *Perceptions of aging in literature: A cross-cultural study*. Westport, CT: Greenwood Press.

Beachamp, T. L., & Childress, J. F. (1989). *Principles of biomedical ethics*. New York: Oxford University Press.

Blazer, D. (1990). *Emotional problems in later life: Intervention strategies for professional caregivers*. New York: Springer.

Foucault, M. (1965). *Madness and civilization*. New York: Vintage.

Fiedler, L. A. (1985). The tyranny of the normal. In T. H. Murray & A. L. Caplan (Eds.), *Which babies shall live? Humanistic dimensions of the care of imperiled newborns* (pp. 151–159). Clifton, NJ: Humana Press.

Grau, L. (Ed.). (1989). *Women in later years: Health, social, and cultural perspectives*. New York: Haworth Press.

Olsen, T. (1961). *Tell me a riddle*. New York: Bantam, Doubleday, Dell.

Spar, J. E., & LaRue, A. (1990). *Geriatric psychiatry*. Washington, DC: American Psychiatric Press.

Waymack, M. H., & Taler, G. A. (1988). *Medical ethics and the elderly: A case book*. Chicago: Pluribus Press.

Yahnke, R. E., & Eastman, R. M. (1990). *Aging in literature: A reader's guide*. Chicago: American Library Association.

VIEW FROM THE FIELD

Perspective From Delaware

■

Mary Lou Hartland

When thinking about the prospect of making comments on a case study in the shadow of giants in the field of ethics I shuddered. How could I possibly add anything that could compare with the impressive commentaries already made by those who are held in such high regard?

I reluctantly read the case studies. I was relieved. I was going to be fine. Why? Because I know these people. I've known them for years.

I knew these clients when I was a case manager. I remembered lying in bed mulling the case over and over trying to make things better, to help, to do the right thing.

These same clients were around when I was a case manager supervisor. I remember them because the case managers would come to me asking for my advice on "the right thing to do."

Now that I am the statewide administrator, one would think that these clients wouldn't be able to find me. Oh no! I travel up and down the small state of Delaware, and they are still with me. Perhaps it isn't Mrs. A or Mr. H, but it is another older person with many of the same perplexing problems. Just as in years past, the answers are still illusive. Making a decision regarding a multifaceted case involving an eccentric, "not-so-rich or famous" person is no easier now than it was then.

Our agency deals with situations like the Mrs. A or Mr. H case regularly. Indeed they are hard to deal with, and there are not clear-cut answers.

The rules listed subsequently are derived from this cumulative experience.

1. Often case managers find themselves struggling with a case in which the issue of eccentricity versus mental illness rears its troublesome head. Deviation from the conventional, the norm, or what is expected is surely different from mental illness. What is relevant or important to the case manager is the degree of risk that the client may be facing. If indeed the older person understands the consequences of their "risky behavior" and makes what is considered to be a bad decision, the case manager must allow the client to be autonomous in his or her decision making.

2. Encouraging a formal competency determination should be done with great care. Forging down such a path without consideration of a person's life-style choices and past history is certainly dangerous territory unless the case manager has clear evidence that the client's competency is in question.

3. A poor score on a canned short mental status questionnaire is not enough to pursue a competency determination. More important is the person's ability to react appropriately in a life-threatening emergency or showing some sense of self preservation. This should certainly carry far greater weight.

4. Forcing someone into the maze of medical and legal realms without strong evidence of lack of competence would be an invasion of the person's autonomy, a direct assault of their dignity, and fall into a gray area in terms of ethical case management.

5. The case manager first and foremost must be an advocate for the client. As an advocate one can do great harm in further alienating members of the community if this action is not pursued in a sensitive manner.

6. Often case managers must take the tactic of being a mediator between their client and the community. Perhaps a plan can be devised to allow the client to remain in the community if a certain degree of compromise can be met.

7. It certainly should be the role of a social service agency to provide education to the community. When the community is well informed and has a heightened sense of awareness regarding individuals' rights to choices in life-style, it is easier to come to some compromise.

8. Clients often live on the edge with the risks being many. To what extent should the case manager determine what risks a client can incur? Clearly, the case manager should only make the determination when the client does not comprehend the consequences of such risk, regardless of what the risk may be.

9. A case manager has the obligation to stick with it, "tough it out," and "hang in there," as long as the client is in agreement with the

care plan. Every avenue should be explored but only if the client is in agreement. A care plan, no matter how ingenious or creative, will never come to fruition unless the client feels that he has had input.

Substandard living conditions, alcohol problems, and so on can only be corrected with the cooperation of the client. That is not to say that the case manager closes the case at the first sign of noncompliance. Many cases take hours of work before a client may be willing to agree to any intervention.

When do case managers end their involvement? This is another good question, but fortunately not on my list. It seems that a case should be closed when case managers can feel confident that they have done everything possible to meet the clients' needs in accordance with the clients' wishes.

EDITORS' QUESTIONS FOR FURTHER DISCUSSION

■

1. Is the distinction between eccentricity and mental illness possible or relevant for case managers?
2. Under what circumstances should a case manager encourage a formal competency determination?
3. How should community sensibilities or community outrage influence the case-management program?
4. To what extent should the case manager determine the risks clients can incur?
5. Once a case manager is involved, is he or she obligated to try to correct substandard living conditions, alcohol problems, and so on?

Chapter 7

FAULT LINES: Boundaries of Abuse and Exploitation

CASE

■

Case managers get into the middle of extraordinarily complicated situations in which they cannot possibly meet the demands that come in from all sides—from the client, from family members, from agencies, from the community, and even from their own agency.

For example, consider a 79-year-old woman with diabetes and circulatory problems. She was physically abused by her daughter with whom she lived and sought assistance from the case manager to get to a safe place. The case manager arranged a group home. She found these arrangements difficult to undertake while respecting everyone's privacy. The client had to see a doctor before she went to the group home, and the doctor noticed the bruises and wanted to know details. The case manager contacted the client's sister who lived in town at the client's request, and, thus, she became involved. A son who lived out of town got involved on his own initiative. Advocates for the elderly got involved through the sister and wanted to place a restraining order on the abusing daughter. Then the courts became involved, and by that time the group home staff wanted to know what was going on.

In all of this, the case manager had difficulty in really tapping the client's preferences, exacerbated because the client was very hard of hearing. The case manager would continually ask her "do you want me to talk to so and so?" or "should I tell so and so about this?" but really the agency was guiding the client through the situation. The case manager thought this client was competent because her responses were appropriate, and she knew what was going on when she could hear. The attorney, whom the case manager found for her and her sister, thought she was competent. Others did not, including other family members and the case manager's supervisor, who thought a guardian was needed. During the hearing about the restraining order, the judge made a speech from the bench about how everyone takes advantage of old people and illustrated with a situation in his own family. He did not grant a restraining order or appoint a guardian at that time.

The client is now deceased. She fell in the group home and had a stroke. She was admitted to a nursing home, and a guardian was then appointed. After her death, the family launched a law suit against the agency, saying that they had mismanaged the case by referring to a group home, which (in contrast to a nursing home) was not equipped to give the client the amount of care she needed. It seemed ironic because the agency had intervened at the client's request to get her away from a daughter who was harming her. In retrospect, the case manager says she thinks she acted correctly, and that the client was enjoying the group home until she fell and had the stroke.

The case manager indicated that she has a difficult time with attorneys in general. With elder abuse situations, she encounters "attorneys who make their livelihood training the states of early dementia people. They probably look at us as bleeding hearts, but we look at them as crooks." For example, one attorney charged $24,000 for guardianship fees in 2 years, though his only work was limited to writing an average of a check a month. The judge called him to court to justify the hourly rates. He relinquished guardianship, but first charged her estate $800 for the morning in court. "It is burglary and robbery, but they don't use a gun." Meanwhile, they needed to find someone else to be the guardian.

Abuse cases are not always clearcut, especially when financial exploitation is at stake. The case manager has a case now in which the client's Social Security check is the only regular income in the home, and her son and his family depend on it. The client is only "sometimes competent," but she is adamant that she wants to stay in that home. The family is on the neglectful side, but they say they love their mother and want her with them. The case manager believes the woman could get better care in a nursing home and that a case of financial exploitation and neglect could be made. But should it be?

COMMENTARIES

Abused or Neglected Clients—or Abusive or Neglectful Service Systems?[1]

■

Adrienne Asch

As I read the material about case management and then read the various hypothetical cases on which we would be asked to comment, I thought of my previous life as a social worker and appreciated that it was a previous life. I probably would rather think about ethical issues than handle some of them, especially if following my conscience might mean losing my job. Quite a number of the cases intrigued me and felt like the best of moral brainteasers.

At first I believed that in the cases here involving physical abuse and financial exploitation, the difficulties lay with the limitations of the individual case manager and not with the system in which he or she operated. By contrast, I believed that where the issue was guardianship appointment and fees, the system, and not the case manager, was at fault. On reflection, I believe that the case manager's personal limitations exacerbate problems in the three vignettes, but that there are pervasive, more intractable systemic problems presented by all three situations. They all concern the social implications of providing assistance to people who need it.

I focus here on two themes that emerge in the three examples: the capacity of individuals to express their wishes and have those wishes heeded, and the desirable relationship between familial and societal obligations to people who need certain types of help. The three individuals who need the help, and who thus come under the system of case management, differ in their capacity to direct how and by whom assistance is provided. Yet the individuals and the institutions that make the arrangements do not adequately recognize and honor such client differences.

GUARDIANSHIP SYSTEM

In the second situation presented, the client has been declared in need of a legal guardian and is presumed to have no decisional capacity. A

---

[1]The author thanks Tamaara Danish, Valentine Doyle, Jill Mazza, and Michael Rozycki for useful suggestions that have improved this discussion.

question not raised, but one that should have been raised, is: How much guardianship does this woman need? In what situations can she not make decisions? Do they encompass all areas of her life, for example, health care, where she lives, and what to do with her money? How much effort has been made to determine her preferences? Needing guardianship in one area, such as handling money, does not imply total incapacity to voice her desires about where she lives, with whom she spends her time, and what medical interventions she receives or refuses.

A second question, also not directly addressed, is that of who should provide assistance in making life decisions if she cannot make them herself. Apparently no family member or friend has been identified as willing or able to assist. The solution is a private attorney who is appointed to serve as guardian. I would suggest that a governmental agency, and not a private attorney, should take on such a responsibility. The state office could then be responsible for regulating both the methods of handling duties and the fees received for them.

The explicit question presented, the case manager's indignation and distress at the behavior of attorneys who serve as guardians and receive high fees for minimal services, is truly only the most blatant problem of an inadequate system of helping people. It is easy to sympathize with the case manager's view that some attorneys are engaging in unacceptable behavior when they charge substantial fees for minimal activity on their ward's behalf. The problem is not merely the profit motives of attorneys; it lies with the society that has not grappled forthrightly with questions of how to provide help for people who need it.

During my work with the New Jersey Bioethics Commission, I discovered a system that avoids at least the financial abuse of individuals by private attorneys, and that also appears to have potential for providing fair, respectful assistance to people who need it. The New Jersey Office of the Public Guardian assumes responsibility for people who are 60 years of age or more, who have been declared incompetent by a court, and who have no friend or family member able to take on legal and decisional authority (New Jersey Commission on Legal and Ethical Problems in the Delivery of Health Care, 1990). Without claiming that the New Jersey system is a model arrangement, it is the stimulus for the system I propose here.

For individuals who have been declared incompetent by a court, and who have not named a proxy decision maker, I propose that a state agency—perhaps the same one that provides case management—should assume legal guardianship. This office should regulate fees for each type of service it performs: x amount for monthly financial transactions; y amount for arranging for social services; and z amount for negotiating medical treatment decisions with physicians. Fees should come from client resources, whether private assets or health insurance, or their entitlements to Medicare or Medicaid. If a public agency assumed guardianship, its own staff could perform the duties, or it could pay the regulated fees to private attorneys. If private attorneys worked under a regulated fee structure, and if a public agency to which they were accountable monitored their services, some of the case manager's problem would be resolved. At least the case manager would not have the conviction that lawyers who act as guardians are robbing the clients (or the state), using expertise instead of more conventional weapons.

Of course, regulating fees for guardianship services would not address such matters as the types of services provided, the qualifications of people providing them, or the methods of assuring that guardians ascertain and respect client preferences. Ideally, social service agencies should persuade their clients to designate someone as a prospective legal guardian. If clients do not wish to name any particular person, they should have the opportunity to register their preference for a public guardian.

As Kathy Powderly suggested during conference discussion (personal communication, July 12, 1991), whenever possible, client designation of a guardianship preference should be accompanied by statements of wishes regarding medical treatment, personal assistance, and finances. Such statements would include information about conditions for which people would and would not be tolerant of treatment; types of medical interventions they would want to receive or to forego; people who should make decisions for them about their medical care; and people who should be entrusted to handle their money for them. Such statements should also include how they want to make tradeoffs: Do they prefer help that might be of lower quality but keeps them in their own home, or does location not matter as much as other factors? Is it more important that assistance be provided by someone they know, even if there is less of it, than by people they have not known before who could come more frequently? If government, social, and health agencies took these steps, the case manager might have fewer instances in which either private attorneys or public officials would be handling the financial and personal affairs of incompetent people.

FAMILIES AS CAREGIVERS

The other two situations illustrate some of these tradeoffs and also bring us to the question of family members as providers of personal assistance. In these two instances, the clients live with family members and receive most of their help from those individuals. One client calls on the case manager to remove her from the "care" of an abusive daughter. In the other instance, we learn that the case manager suspects financial exploitation of a mother by her son and his family.

In the first example, a client reported physical abuse at the hands of her daughter and requested a change in her living situation. Although the vignette describes the case manager as anxious and perplexed about the handling of the situation *after* the abuse was reported, the more serious problems are in the adequacy of the initial assessment and not in the ethics of the resolution. The case manager and the employing agency should rethink how they assessed client needs and resources in the first place, considering at least the following questions: Could services provided earlier have prevented an abusive situation from developing between mother and daughter? Should the mother have been helped to recognize that she needed more assistance than her daughter could comfortably provide or that she should live elsewhere? Could case-management services have included relieving the daughter of some physical duties? Or would psychological services for mother and daughter have enabled them to deal with problems in their relationship and thereby have prevented abuse?

Certainly, as either advocate or gatekeeper, the case manager is primarily accountable to the client or to the person acting as decisionmaker for the client, and not to judges or other family members. The client appears to have been alert and capable of participating in many decisions regarding her own life, and it would seem that the worker was accountable to her and her preferences as long as she was able to give opinions. The client recognized and reported abuse and requested that her sister be notified of the situation as it developed. If the worker was uncertain about whether others (the client's son or other professionals) could be involved, the worker should have consulted with the client about which people she was willing to inform. If there was some concern about whether the client could hear and understand her questions, the worker should have presented them in writing. If they had to be spoken, they should have been put to her more than once, in different ways, to assure that she understood and answered them consistently. To do anything less is to make physical incapacity tantamount to complete cognitive incapacity, an unfortunate and all-too-persistent response to dealing with elderly and disabled people (Wright, 1983).

Similarly, the client should have been able to select from a range of options the most appropriate setting in which to live. If the case manager wonders whether the choice of a group home was appropriate, the answer should be found in the client's reaction. Did the client know of other options and choose it in preference to such facilities as a nursing home? Did the client understand the level of help she required, or the level she would get in different settings? If so, and if the client chose the group setting in which she fell, the case manager can feel that the decision was made responsibly. Who is to know that the client might not have fallen in another setting or in her own home—perhaps fleeing from an abusive action of her daughter?

Less clear is the last example of possible financial abuse of a client by a son. Yet, there is reason to question the case manager's characterization of a woman being taken advantage of financially by her relatives. What is the neglect described in the sentence "the family is on the neglectful side"? What does the worker mean by "care"? Does she mean that the mother would be more cared about, or better cared for? Would the "care" be better in another setting if the son and his mother want to live together?

Exactly what makes the worker think that the woman is being financially exploited? Is she deprived of things she wants because the son's family is using the money without consulting her? Before reporting exploitation as abuse, it would make more sense for the worker to reassess the help the client needs and receives, the relationship of provider to client, and the client's preferences. Even if the client is only "sometimes competent," such a description tells little. Competent how often? Competent to say what? Competent to recognize what situations? A client may be unable to decide how to spend her money but quite capable of recognizing when she is being given affection and attention that is satisfying. Such attention and affection may be more important to the client than possible misallocation of money. And during the client's competent moments, why not find out whether she has desires about the use of her money that are being ignored? If so, there is a potential problem that needs intrafamily communication (perhaps with the help of the case manager), and not reporting to an external agency. If there is no such client dissatisfaction, the case manager might better worry about the system's financial exploitation of clients by profit-seeking lawyers than by hard-pressed relatives who give physical help and love.

CHANGE OF SYSTEM

Thus far, my comments on the instances of physical abuse and financial exploitation have been limited to the case manager operating within the existing system of policy and service for people who need assistance. A genuinely satisfactory resolution for the two women clients requires altering this system to permit addressing separately what assistance is needed, who will direct its provision, which people should provide it, and in what setting it should be provided. At issue is our understanding of the status of people who need assistance, and how, where, and by whom people who need certain types of help should obtain it.

Underlying all that follows is the assumption made about the status of the person who receives the help, generally termed "care." Two connotations of "care" lead to the difficulties inherent in the existing system. The first connotation diminishes the status of the person who receives assistance; the second causes people to confuse and inappropriately combine the activities of helping someone and having warmth and affection for that person.

Think of the difference between the words "help" and "care." Someone whose car stops on the highway may ask a passing motorist for help, such as to change a flat tire, go for gas, or call the police. The individual who needs something at one time might be the person who provides something else at another time, perhaps to the motorist, perhaps to someone else. "Care" connotes an asymmetrical relationship in which someone who needs all-encompassing help receives it from another, who is more capable in all areas. By using the phrase "long-term care," I believe that professionals and family members unwittingly, without realizing that they have done so, accord a lesser social position to the person who needs help simply because she or he has this need. Task-specific assistance is not global care. Needing help with toileting, dressing, and cooking implies nothing about needing help to make decisions about what to do with one's time, money, or friends and relatives. Among the first changes needed in the field of "long-term care" is new language to replace "care" with "assistance" or "help," reflecting the understanding that needing help in some areas is not equivalent to being incapable in all areas.

The term "care" also connotes having concern for, or "caring about," as in "have warm feelings for" the other person. All too often, professional discussion of the needs of people with any activity-limiting condition assumes that the individual will receive this help, termed "care," from a family member. Family assistance is favored as an alternative to socially provided care based first on cost and second on its presumed buttressing of values of kinship and the duties that go with kinship. The assumption is that only as a last resort should such "care" be provided by others, either paid workers who come to the home, or paid workers who help people in group or institutional settings.

I challenge just this assumption and propose that assistance with activities of daily living, no matter what and how much assistance, might best be provided by people who are *not* family members. To assist someone is not to take care of or to care about another person. Assistance need not be provided as part of a loving or ostensibly loving relationship.

Sometimes people who need help with dressing, bathing, shopping, cooking, or the like will prefer to receive this help from those they know and love, and their loved ones will comfortably incorporate giving this assistance into a mutually fulfilling relationship. At their best, loving friendships or family relationships include willingness to help people in various ways—sometimes physical, sometimes financial, sometimes emotional. In a comfortable relationship, the daughter who helps her mother get dressed also benefits from her mother's companionship and the sharing of pleasurable activities. What professionals forget, but fortunately what many families remember, is that the one who can no longer manage certain physical tasks still has other ways to contribute to family life. Ideally, people can incorporate providing and receiving assistance into their relationship without one person's feeling burdened and the other's feeling guilty. However, even excellent relationships can be marred if one person feels that she is being asked to do more than she can manage comfortably, as Callahan (1988) points out in an article quite representative in its portrayal of the harm that helping a disabled family member can do to the lives of the others in the family.

There is no necessary connection between loving a parent, sibling, or spouse and providing such help. In fact, I would argue that separating the provision of such assistance from other personal relationships may preserve the dignity and privacy of the person requiring the help and the mutuality of intimate relationships.

Many people with disabilities who need assistance with housekeeping, dressing, eating, hygiene, reading, or communicating go to considerable lengths to purchase those services rather than receive them from friends or family. They believe that services to maintain life or to permit them to function in the world at a level comparable with those without disabilities are not services that have anything to do with the essence of intimate relationships. What many disabled people want in their friends and loved ones is the companionship and emotional closeness that everyone else wants. They may prefer to receive instrumental help from people with whom they are not closely emotionally involved to ensure that they and their loved ones retain the time, the equality, and the reciprocity to enjoy what is intrinsic to the personal relationship.

Whether people with disabilities are young or old, or live alone or with others, they all might be better off if they could count on having the option to obtain reliable help with life-maintaining activities from people who specifically elect to take on these tasks (Crewe & Zola, 1983; Litvak, Zukas, & Heumann, 1987). If the physically abused or financially exploited mothers could have received reliable assistance from others, they might well have preferred to live apart from their children. Conversely, living with their children might have been easier for them, as well as their children, had it been acceptable for people to come into a home to help with dressing or shopping, in the same way that it is acceptable to need and hire carpenters, plumbers, tutors, or housekeepers.

As adults, it is hoped that people associate with one another because they wish to do so, not because they must. Writing from the perspective of the grown child considering an aging parent, Jane English (1979) points out that the grown child should not have to feel that former parental sacrifices require particular responses. Her point is that, ideally, grown children will choose to spend time with and help their parents because they appreciate and enjoy them as people, perhaps including appreciation of what those people did for them when they were children.

The same can be said from the standpoint of the older person who is the typical client of case managers in long-term care programs. Neither outmoded equating of impairment with total incapacity, nor inadequate social arrangements should trap the client into living with or taking help from relatives or friends. If the cardinal rule of case management is to respect client preferences (Kane, 1990), case managers and their agencies should work to create a system that respects client autonomy in something as basic as freedom of association. By separating a need for certain assistance from the expectation that family members should render it, a service system could permit people to receive help in some areas without losing control of their own lives. Such a system could also permit clients and their families to rediscover that which is potentially precious and unique in close relationships.

REFERENCES

Callahan, D. (1988, May). Families as caregivers: The limits of morality, *Archives of Physical Medicine and Rehabilitation, 69*, 13–18.

Crewe, N. S., & Zola, I. K. (Eds.). (1983). *Independent living for physically disabled people: Developing, implementing, and evaluating self-help rehabilitation programs.* San Francisco, CA: Jossey-Bass.

English, J. (1979). What do grown children owe their parents? In O. O'Neill & W. Ruddick (Eds.), *Having children: Philosophical and legal reflections on parenthood.* New York: Oxford University Press.

Kane, R. A. (1990). What is case management anyway? In R. A. Kane, E. K. Urv-Wong, & C. King (Eds.), *Case management: What is it anyway?*

Minneapolis, MN: University of Minnesota, Long-Term Care Decisions Resource Center.

Litvak, S., Zukas, H., & Heumann, J. E. (1987). *Attending to America: Personal assistance for independent living.* Berkeley, CA: World Institute on Disability.

New Jersey Commission on Legal and Ethical Problems in the Delivery of Health Care. (1990). *Problems and approaches in health care decisionmaking: The New Jersey experience.* Princeton, NJ: New Jersey Commission on Legal and Ethical Problems in the Delivery of Health Care.

Wright, B. A. (1983). *Physical disability: A psychosocial approach.* New York: Harper & Row.

Values and Perspectives on Abuse: Unspoken Influences on Ethical Reasoning

■

Rebecca Dresser

This "case" presentation actually includes three specific cases that together raise a variety of ethical issues. In essence, I see five general areas that are relevant to the presentation: (a) client competency; (b) the nature of client choice; (c) the definition and reporting of client abuse and neglect; (d) the client's relationship with her family; and (e) the problems inherent in the state system of protecting the client's "best interests." The customary medical ethics code words—autonomy, beneficence, and justice—each have a role in the analysis of these areas. But I would like to go beyond the "Big Three" here, to unpack some of the other values, attitudes, and emotions that will inevitably influence one's beliefs about the appropriate way to respond to cases like these.

First, let me describe some of my reactions to the case descriptions. Before going to law school, I completed a master's degree in counseling. I contemplated social work as a career, and I spent some time working with boys in a juvenile detention center. Then I was a welfare worker for a year. Reading these cases and the other materials describing case management brought back to me some of the feelings I experienced during that time. Most dominant was the frustration I felt in attempting to work within a complex, restrictive bureaucracy that rarely even began to meet my clients' needs. There was also the discouraging sense that by the time the clients got to me, there was little hope that things would ever get much better for them. The vast majority had been born into families with many of the same problems my clients had—poor education, low self-esteem, and other characteristics that left them ill equipped to cope with the harshness and intricacies of contemporary American life. All I could do was give them the little bit permitted by the system I represented. It was too depressing for me—I escaped to law school and sheltered academia. So I approach these cases with a mixture of attitudes: relief at not having to address these problems in my daily working life; sadness at the plight of the clients who struggle with them; and admiration for the case managers and others who can cope with them better than I could.

I have indulged in these personal reflections partly because they will inescapably affect how I look at the cases, but also because I believe it is important for us to look into ourselves when we are asked to react to a situation in someone else's life, whether it is just on paper, as this one is, or in "real life," as the case manager must do (Burt, 1979). In light of this view, I begin by discussing some of the other dimensions of our own experiences that may influence what we see as the "appropriate" way to address these cases. There are no easy answers here, nor are there many absolutes (although we probably can agree on a few). Our differences on what is ethically permissible or required will largely be a function of where we stand and who we are, I think.

ASSESSMENT OF ONE'S OWN VALUES AND PERSPECTIVES

Before the assessment of the client should come the case manager's assessment of herself. The case manager has a responsibility to look at her own moral values and social position. She ought to acknowledge to herself, indeed, perhaps to the client, when these are affecting her judgments concerning the best way to manage a case. "Fault Lines" seems to me to implicate several possible personal perspectives that could influence the case manager's handling of these cases.

ATTITUDES TOWARD FAMILY RESPONSIBILITIES

First is the case manager's views on the obligations and duties family members have to their relatives in need. One client in the description has a daughter who physically abuses her, another has a son who depends on his mother's Social Security check to support his family. Here we have children who seem to be violating even the most minimal ethical obligation—to refrain from inflicting positive harm on others. You shouldn't physically assault or steal from a stranger, much less your mother!

So it's easy to condemn the abusing daughter—but how many of us have lived with an elderly and disabled parent? How many of us would have difficulty living with even a perfectly healthy parent? Perhaps there is a way to intervene to decrease the daughter's stress and still maintain any benefits the client may gain from living with her child. Similarly, our initial reaction to the "embezzling" son is that he is taking unfair advantage of a vulnerable elderly parent, and of us taxpayers as well. So we want to get the "victim" into a place where her interests come first—but where is that? A nursing home?

The way the case manager reacts to the behavior of the adult children will inevitably affect her view of what should happen to the clients in these cases. It will determine whether she takes the time to look further at these problematic home situations to discover if there is a less restrictive alternative than outright removal. On balance, drastic methods that can destroy family ties may be more harmful for clients than what appear to be abysmal home situations. In this culture, most of us are ambivalent about family relationships. We tend to see families as sources of great love and joy, but also as sources of great pain. For case managers, it is important to recognize these feelings in themselves, their clients, and their clients' families. The complexities inherent in family interactions may often call for a more nuanced approach than is apparent on first examination of a client's situation (Minow, 1990).

ATTITUDES TOWARD AGING AND DISABILITY

The case manager's attitudes toward aging and disability will also strongly influence her views of these cases. In all three, elderly and impaired clients are placed at the mercy of their conniving families and lawyer-guardians. It seems these clients ought to be rescued, protected for their own good.

But, again, let us take a closer look. In the first case, there is an abused, "79-year-old woman with diabetes and circulatory problems" who is seeking help in escaping to a safe place. The case manager thinks the client is competent, but communication is difficult because the client is "very hard of hearing." The client's lawyer agrees that the client is competent, but the client's children and the case manager's supervisor claim that a guardian is needed. The judge makes a speech about "how everyone takes advantage of old people" and refuses to name a guardian or grant an order restraining the daughter from having contact with her mother.

Apparently, no one in this case tried very hard to talk to the client. It appears that being very hard of hearing, as well as elderly and beset with medical problems, means that you fade into the background while other people argue about your desires and preferences. On the one hand, we have a woman who was strong enough to assert herself and ask the case manager for assistance. Conversely, we have several people arguing over this "helpless" woman's fate without bothering very much to include her in the discussion. Did anyone think of a hearing aid or some other means of addressing the client's hearing problem? Did anyone think of communicating with her in writing?

In the second case, there is an incompetent client whose estate has been depleted of $24,000 in 2 years by her lawyer-guardian. Here we have a client who was deemed impaired enough to lose control of her wealth but not important enough to be provided a guardian who would adequately protect it for her. In the final case, there is a "sometimes competent" client who adamantly insists that she wants to remain in a home that seems exploitative and neglectful to the case manager.

The cases reveal several commonplace attitudes toward elderly and impaired individuals. First, such individuals often lose their status as full-fledged persons when it becomes too difficult for others to talk with them. Clients like these are excluded from full participation in the world because the customary methods of communication are unavailable to those around them. Instead of facing the communication challenges with creativity, the younger, healthier people simply take over. But assessing competency absolutely requires communication with the client. Competency is a function of a person's ability to understand the choices she is facing, the circumstances relevant to the decision at hand (Appelbaum, Lidz, & Meisel, 1987). If there is a means of communicating with the client, there is an obligation to find and use it before forming judgments on her capacity to participate in decisions.

One's attitudes toward becoming old will also inevitably color one's reaction to the cases. Although the model of old age has changed to some extent, I still think that in our society, becoming old is something most people dread. Images of abandonment, loss of control and respect, physical restriction, financial problems, and so forth come to mind for many of us. The judge in the second case was apparently identifying strongly with the client when he gave his speech about "how everyone takes advantage of old people." These feelings may trigger intense anger toward those who seem to be responsible for mistreating and neglecting their elderly relatives or clients. Often, such a reaction may be entirely justified. It seems important, however, to be aware of when we are reacting to our fears about our own futures rather than to the client's particular situation. The judge in this case "lost" the client—he apparently did not even bother to talk with her. As a result, the judge's decision may have been more responsive to his own needs than to those of the client.

"IDEAL" DECISION MAKING

One's notion of what constitutes "ideal" human decision making will also exert an effect on one's view of cases one and three in "Fault Lines." Are people's choices ideally made completely "free" from external constraints and the undue influence of others? Or is this a rarefied picture of human life that neglects our existence as social beings? Moreover, when does another person's influence over a client's decision become "undue"? Finally, should we conceive of people primarily as autonomous individuals, or as members of a family and community whose choices are inevitably strongly influenced by their environments?

These issues arise most starkly in the third case, in which a "sometimes competent" client is "adamant" about staying in what the case manager sees as an exploitative and neglectful home situation. Here, the case manager seems to characterize the client's decision as a poor one; indeed, the case manager's view that the client is only "sometimes competent" may be affected by her view of the quality of the client's decision. The case manager believes that the client's desire to remain with her son is misguided, that the client's preferences are being improperly manipulated, and that if the client were able to make a "truly free" choice, she would choose to live elsewhere. She would choose, that is, the decision that the case manager herself thinks would be best for the client.

It seems to me that the case manager needs to engage in some soul searching here. There are a multiplicity of factors relevant to the client's decision about where to live. One is, of course, her physical safety and well-being, which may not be receiving enough attention in the son's home. But there are other factors as well. The client's psychological and emotional needs are equally, if not more, important to the client's overall well-being. A nursing home might well provide better physical care to the client. But how well would her other needs be addressed there?

Again, it seems to me that the case manager needs to spend more time talking with her client. A better competency assessment may be needed.

What does the client understand about the choices she has available to her? Does she know what to do if her physical well-being is seriously threatened? Is she capable of speaking up if she is in danger? What is her view of the nursing home? How does she picture her life there?

Furthermore, the case manager should expand her own view of the client's best interests, to consider more than just physical needs. What kinds of contact would the client have with her family if she entered a nursing home? Would the client be likely to form new relationships at the nursing home, or is it more probable that she would become withdrawn in the new situation? Choices like this one are never simple, and no solution will be ideal. The outcome must reflect a balance of the many variables relevant to the choice including the variables the case manager now seems to be neglecting. The client may be making a better choice than the case manager believes. There may also be ways of improving the client's physical care while allowing her to remain in the son's home, for example, by arranging for visiting nurse services or regular home visits by a social worker. The client's choice may be overridden if it places her in serious physical danger. This ought to be a last resort, however, as long as the son's home is providing her with important "services" the nursing home would omit.

GENDER AND CLASS ISSUES

It seems to me that the actions in these three cases were also affected by the gender and economic positions of the players. All of the clients are women; as we all know, a substantial majority of elderly clients are women. The case manager is female, and the embezzling attorney and the judge are male. In our society, there is a tradition of the financially better-off making decisions about how the less well-off will live, and of men making decisions about how women will live. The tradition continues, as is obvious in these cases. Moreover, the case manager is fulfilling the time-honored tradition of working in one of the low-paid, low-status "caring" professions that women have tended to enter, whereas the high-paid, high-status positions are occupied by men. Meanwhile, there are three women who need the "care and protection" of the largely male legal system.

These social realities most clearly surface in case two. The case manager "has a difficult time with attorneys in general" and cites as an example a lawyer-guardian who obviously overcharged for his services. Although he was eventually dismissed, he apparently was not penalized for this behavior. The case manager feels powerless to protect her clients' interests when she must operate in a system like this. Her reaction is quite understandable. It is a bad system. The question is how best to deal with its flaws. Better guardians are certainly one answer. This is an area in which case managers may need to look beyond their individual clients and attempt to institute systemwide improvement. Many courts would probably welcome assistance in developing improvements in the process for selecting guardians. In addition, when the case manager observes what she believes to be improper conduct by a guardian, she ought to report it. Passivity only strengthens the unfairness and inadequacy of the existing system.

CONCLUSION

In this analysis, I have tried to get away from the typical "ethicist" approach, and instead, to discuss some of the underlying, usually unspoken influences on one's view of the "best" ethical outcome in a difficult case. I know that I have not addressed every issue, of course. I do hope, however, that my approach has fostered consideration of these cases and the issues they raise from a deeper and more expansive perspective. It is often as important to examine the viewer's situation as it is to examine the situation of the person being "viewed." In light of the huge impact case managers may have on their clients' lives, it seems particularly important to do so in this area.

REFERENCES

Appelbaum, P., Lidz, T., & Meisel, A. (1987). *Informed consent: Legal theory and clinical practice.* New York: Oxford University Press.
Burt, R. (1979). *Taking care of strangers.* New York: Free Press.
Minow, M. (1990). *Making all the difference: Inclusion, exclusion, and American law.* Ithaca, NY: Cornell University Press.

VIEW FROM THE FIELD

Perspective From Pennsylvania

■

Richard Browdie

Having been asked for my personal reaction to the case offered, the following represents my individual reflections as an administrator who has seen these issues at the state and local levels.

From a moral viewpoint, the case manager can be viewed as being accountable to virtually everybody. But as a practical matter, most case managers are accountable first to the agencies they work for. From there, most would like to view themselves as being accountable to clients and to any laws or regulations that control their behavior. Certainly when a court chooses to intervene, the case worker can be held accountable to a judge, but by the time that has happened, most of the dilemmas will have been resolved.

The difficulty presented by the first case is associated with the conflicting opinions regarding the woman's competence, and conflicting values regarding appropriate care and living arrangements. If competent, adults can decide to do things that seem ill advised and dangerous. But if their competence is being evaluated solely on the basis of an observer's judgment of the appropriateness of the decision, we may slide into using our own values as a determinant of what people should be allowed to do.

This is a particularly thorny issue for public agency case managers, because case managers, particularly if they happen to gain the interest of an elected official, can bring a great deal of force to bear on a client or a family to encourage their cooperation. And, in fact, a great deal of pressure can be brought to bear on the public official, who has control over an agency that can intervene when so directed. Clients whose situations offend "community standards" are at risk of being "railroaded" into solutions that they don't want because someone else knows better what they need and should want.

One of the most difficult areas to assess is family relationships and when interdependence is transcended by abuse. In most states, there are abuse-reporting systems that workers would be expected to use. Indeed, the worker would be in a good position to try to differentiate between abuse and interdependence before coming to the conclusion that abuse was present. The difficult task of knowing when it has crossed the line is made even more difficult by the complications common to family relationships. Conflict may be an important part of the relationship, and fighting may be "normal" in a family. If a client is in all other ways competent and seems to want to stay in a situation that seems uncomfortable to us, we would be hard-pressed to find any justification to intervene except for our own values. In fact, family relationships of all types are probably not an appropriate area for case managers to be involved except when there is some observable negative impact on the client. And then, their concern has to be directed to only resolving issues that are relevant to the client's well-being.

This leads to probably the most difficult of the questions posed. Can a presumably competent client choose to be exploited or harmed? The only way that the answer could be no is if the client can be compelled to take steps that meet someone else's criteria for appropriateness. If a client chooses to live in an environment that seems unsafe, even just not as "good" as another environment, the decision has to be made as to whose values will prevail. So long as the client is competent, it must be his or her values. And if the client's competence is in question, then it has to be tested by whatever standards prevail before the case manager or agency, or community for that matter, can impose its will.

Even financial exploitation versus interdependence or "sharing of resources" requires a value judgment to be made. Exploitation implies coercion or some sort of fraudulent misdirection of resources. But response to the problems of others can be as important to an older person as their own needs. Willing and unwilling sacrifices are made among families all the time. When it becomes clear that the client is unwilling or is unknowingly being exploited, then it can be differentiated from interdependence. But when it arrives at that point is a matter of judgment, and, again, a competent older person is the best judge of his or her own interests.

EDITORS' QUESTIONS FOR FURTHER DISCUSSION

■

1. To whom are case managers accountable? Clients? Family? Guardians? Judges? Anyone else?
2. Whom should case managers notify if they suspect abuse, neglect, or exploitation?
3. To what extent are family relationships case managers' business?
4. Can we distinguish between a family's financial interdependence and financial exploitation?
5. Can clients choose to be exploited or harmed by others?

Chapter 8

FINAL PLACEMENTS: Home or Nursing Home?

CASE

■

Two sisters live together. One is blind and the other has advanced pulmonary disease. The latter sister, Miss E, needs a lot of care, and her sister cannot give it well though she is willing to continue trying. The program can pay for 4 hours of help a day, but the case manager thinks this is inadequate. She doubts either sister really gets enough to eat and sees the house has become run down. Miss E has emphysema and is hospitalized with an attack of asthma. She is determined to go back home, but everyone gangs up and persuades her to try a nursing home. Within 4 days, she is dead. The case manager is sure the change of place and the trauma of moving to the nursing home hastened her death. She felt terrible—she felt she had killed her. Does this result suggest nobody should have interfered with Miss E's plan to go home?

The case manager is perturbed by this case, which unfortunately seems to be a variation of many of her cases. Often family members push for nursing home care because they don't want to help enough, or because they are just so worried. The case manager sometimes sees their point. But some clients do need much more care than they can get at home. She has a client with multiple sclerosis who is moved from bed to a chair and left alone all day to sit in her wastes. She is alone for 8 hours at a time. Yet this very same client wants to stay at home despite these disadvantages.

She also had a client—a man with an unstable heart condition and mobility problems—whom she helped persuade to give in to family wishes and try a nursing home. After a few days he asked the case manager to help him get out of there. His apartment was gone, but she did find other housing. But in the few days that it took to arrange this, the man changed his mind again. The doctor had been in and convinced him that he should not be trying to live alone at his age. Within a few weeks after that, the man was also dead.

The case manager wonders what to make of these examples of death shortly after nursing home admission. With the man with the heart condition, "I felt as though I had killed him." But the case manager is aware that one of her colleagues found a client dead at home last year. Not only is her case-manager colleague still in shock, but the family is suing the case manager and the agency for an inadequate care plan. They always thought their dad should have been in a nursing home. The case manager figures you are "damned if you do and damned if you don't." Certainly her colleague is thinking twice now whenever she leaves someone at home with a flimsy care plan.

One thing the case manager feels strongly about is the person with a physical condition who plans to die at home. She thinks this is okay. She has watched people make that choice and even slowly stop eating. The problem is that once they become confused, which they are bound to do as they near death, their wish is not respected, and they end up dying in a nursing home or hospital. The case manager thinks that isn't right, though one of her colleagues says, "what does it matter?" The client is getting comfort care, the family is relieved, and the client doesn't know where she is anyway.

COMMENTARIES

Can the Case Manager Offer Placement in Good Conscience?

■

Arthur L. Caplan

Case managers are no less immune to magical thinking, fantasy, and guilt then anyone else. I have asked many health care professionals with expertise in psychiatry, psychology, and the behavioral sciences, including many with significant experience in dealing with the elderly, about the claim that moving a patient from one setting to another, even permanently, can result in death. Every one of them without exception rejected the claim that any evidence exists that supports the view that moving a patient from one setting to another, changing the environment in which they live and receive care, poses a lethal risk or can be implicated as a cause of a person's death. The only exception mentioned by these health care professionals was that there do exist some obvious risk factors that can be exacerbated by physical movement.

Many elderly people with severe pulmonary disease will die. Some of these patients, such as Miss E, die when they are moved from home to nursing home, home to ambulance, nursing home to hospital, or hospital to hospice. They die, not because their setting is changed, but, because they are old, frail, and suffering from a life-threatening disease.

There is some data to support the claim that older people tend to live until they have reached dates which represent or connote significant events in their lives such as an anniversary, a birthday, or a religious holiday. But there is no evidence that moving someone from one place to another, even permanently, is lethal. It may be stressful. It certainly can be depressing. But, changing settings, even against a person's wishes or desires, is not a murderous act.

So why then is the case manager so troubled about and convinced that moving Miss E from home to nursing home resulted in her death 4 days later? The case worker's concerns about changing settings are not confined to the case of Miss E. Apparently the case worker thinks that many patients die as a result of involuntary transfers from home to nursing home. Yet, the case manager must also know as well as anyone else can that actuarial charts do not paint a cheery picture for elderly persons who are in advanced stages of lung, heart or liver disease. Some who are as ill as Miss E are going to die within the next 4 days no matter whether they remain still and immobile or are driven to a new location every night. The law of large numbers means that some elderly patients with severe emphysema or COPD are going to die within the next week or two whether they go to the nursing home with a smile on their face and a sigh of relief at finally being able to be away from the kids or spitting in the eye of the bastards who sent them to the hellhole that now must be called home.

So what is going on? Why are so many case managers (and not a few families) so certain that they have killed some of their clients by making them go where they did no want to go? What is going on in terms of the beliefs of case managers is more a function of the gap that exists between ideals and reality than it is geography, institutions, and environment.

Most people do not want to go to nursing homes. They hate them. They fear them. Every adult whom I have ever heard describe the decision to send a parent to a nursing home has done so with the firm conviction that, in doing so, they are conducting the secular equivalent of the ritual engaged in by some Inuit peoples of sending their frail elderly out to certain death on an icefloe. Case managers know all about these attitudes. Moreover, they know that the dread of nursing homes so endemic in our society is not entirely without a basis in reality. The conditions that prevail in too many nursing homes are not only not conducive to autonomy, they are not conducive to safety, sanity, or familiarity.

Why do people want to stay in their own homes? People want to stay home because they like familiar surroundings, familiar smells, familiar memories. They do not like going to other places to live for the same reason that almost no one likes to do without these familiar experiences.

Familiarity does not breed contempt when it comes to where we live. Familiarity breeds peace of mind because we feel safe and secure in environments that we have helped to shape and that reflect our emotional and psychological handiwork.

I hate staying in hotels. I can never figure out how to turn on the heat or the air conditioning. I do not have this problem in my own house because I know where the controls are for the thermostat. I would not like the nursing home because not only could I not find the controls, but I also might not be able to alter them if the building had central heat. Shifting persons who have established long histories with their environments to new environments may not literally kill them, but it may so imperil their sense of the familiar that they feel a complete loss of control and autonomy.

Nursing homes permit little familiarity. They are institutions that keep an eye on their budgets, as well as the overall well-being of their residents and their functional stability. This is not so much a malicious or evil thing to do as it is a quintessentially bureaucratic thing to do. Nursing homes are not hospitable to the familiar not because no one who works there cares, but because what makes places familiar to persons is that they have the opportunity to interact with and shape them so that they reflect a tiny bit of themselves. It is next to impossible to do this in the Spartan, controlled, and communally oriented environment of the nursing home.

Why don't hospitals engender the same dread images? Well, to be honest for many people they do. But I suspect that the fear of the hospital is lessoned by the realization of those who face going there that they do not have to live there. Nursing homes are places people go to live; hospitals are places people go for a time to get better. Hospitals are never seen as homes, but, as some recent research done at Minnesota shows, nursing homes are often seen as permanent abodes. And homes should be familiar.

Sending Gramps to the home is to be dreaded because Gramps is headed to a place where the exile is irreversible, communication sporadic, the food bland, and the lights go off when the rules say they must. Gramps cannot shape the environment of the place where he is being sent to live, and he will not feel any tie of familiarity with his new surroundings.

Ironically, contrary to the worry of the sort expressed by Miss E's case manager, the lack of familiarity is unlikely to kill him, especially because he will be dwelling in a location that has nurses and nurses aides available in a way that is not true about individual homes. If Gramps or Miss E have respiratory arrests they are more at risk of winding up with a nasogastric tube and a vent then they would be if they were allowed to stay at home or with their relatives or children. But those who go to nursing homes are not likely to feel kindly toward their new institutional home, and everyone who visits will know that this is so.

Case managers know that nursing homes are not hotbeds of individuality and personal choice. They also know very well that they are obligated to present all options for living environments to their competent clients and to their surrogate decision makers if their clients' competency is impaired or variable. They understand that respect for the autonomy and the dignity of the client obligates them to maximize client options, explain the risks and benefits associated with each choice, and to work with clients and their families to make sure that coercion is absent and voluntariness undergirds all placement decisions.

But, case managers know that there is a big gap between the ideal of informed consent and the real world of options. If the goal of case management with respect to placement is to maximize the freedom enjoyed by clients by eliminating restrictions and obstacles to choice in the environment where the client will live, and maximize the opportunities and range of options available to their clients, then informed consent can be something of a cruel hoax when the placements choices are restrictive and full of obstacles, and the range of options is narrow. Nursing homes rarely do much for the enhancement of positive freedom, such as creating options, opportunities, and choices; instead they often are settings in which negative freedom including interference, intrusions, restraints, and restrictions flourish.

Not only are case managers, often in cahoots with families, sending their clients to institutions that are not and, as they are currently structured, cannot be concerned with the creation of familiarity and individuality, or positive freedom, but, their clients must be sent there with their voluntary, informed consent. Yet, most clients cannot really exercise even a semblance of autonomy about where they will spend their final days because such decisions are often fraught with coercion and fiscal pressures. Offering options that may not exist to those who lack the means, the resources, and the financial and psychological capacities to act on them is cruel. Better to diminish the guilt engendered by a close inspection of the gap between what professional duty requires in the name of client consent and what reality offers in the way of constrained, limited, and tightly controlled communal environments by embracing the belief that clients ought to be sent to nursing homes because their lives hang in the balance.

Patient choice, ideally, should determine placement for any competent patient. But the system that exists for long-term care is neither a system nor does it exist. The sole determinant for the case manager in thinking about placement for a competent client is what placement is most likely to maximize positive freedom for the client and to minimize encroachments on negative freedom. When the client is not competent, then the moral dilemma becomes trying to decide whether infringements on negative freedom that enhance the chance of positive freedom are acceptable and who is in the best position to make that judgment. Presuming families to be in the best position to make the call seems reasonable. Presuming the value of accepting restrictions on negative freedom, the right to be left alone, if balanced by corresponding increases in positive freedom, the right to do more and to have greater choice seems reasonable as well. But neither rule seems reasonable if the only options available are unlikely to permit the individuality and thus the familiarity and freedom that makes life worthwhile in one's home.

Are nursing home placements categorically bad? The answer is for most of them yes. The litmus test is whether they are constructed and organized so as to permit the individuality that would allow residents to feel at home in them, to find the nursing home or make the nursing home a familiar place. Most institutions fail this test.

Can the case manager offer the option of placement in good conscience knowing this is so? Probably not, though the powerful, persistent myth of death by nursing home placement is more reflective of the fallacy of seeking consent to a place where no one would reasonably want to go than it is a realistic account of why elderly frail persons die when they are moved.

Death and the Case Manager

■

Rebecca Elon

The reaction of the case manager to the death of a client is a theme running through the case scenarios presented here. Although it may seem heretical to say in some circles and unnecessary to say in others, death is an inevitable and natural part of life. The clients often know this better than do the professionals. When dealing with a very frail elderly population of clients, case managers will be working within the terminal phase of life for many of the people they serve. How the case manager deals with and reacts to the deaths of clients is an issue that may be directly related to the professional longevity of the case manager in working with this population.

There is profound sadness and grieving at the loss of someone with whom a professional relationship, and perhaps a fondness, has been established. There is guilt and self-doubt that "perhaps I hastened this death through an act or omission." There is shock when "I walked in and found her dead." There is fear because "perhaps I will be sued for the way I handled this case which ended with the death of the client."

It is imperative for case managers to create a means and mechanism within their work environment for open discussion with colleagues about difficult cases, for periodic review and assessment of professional performance, for continuing education, for mutual support, for learning from mistakes, and, at times, for absolution. The work demands it. Without it, burnout and dropout rates will be high as case managers ridden with grief, guilt, self-doubt, and fear leave the field for brighter, more rewarding endeavors.

If the focus of one's work is prolongation of life, and death is always considered the enemy, the case manager serving a frail elderly popula-tion will become weary of repeatedly losing the battles and will finally abandon the unwinable war. In assessing professional performance in cases that end with the death of the client, what guideposts can the case manager use to decide whether the best possible care was given or whether changes in approach should be pursued in future similar cases? When is death a good outcome, or a neutral outcome, as opposed to an exclusively bad outcome? Because the occurrence of death may accom-pany excellent care or substandard care, what elements of the process of care can be of assistance in judging professional performance?

One essential component within the process of care is enhancing the client's sense of control over the situation. Taking control away from frail elderly clients may not only violate their right to self-determination, but may also profoundly affect their emotional and physical health (Rodin, 1986). It has been demonstrated that undesirable events over which an individual has full control correlate with no change in a measured index of strain, whereas undesirable events over which the individual has no control strongly correlate with strain (Rowe & Kahn, 1987). Although the literature on morbidity and mortality associated with relocation of the elderly is plagued with methodological problems, multiple studies on the effects of involuntary relocation and in-stitutionalization of the elderly exist (Kasl, 1972). There are studies demonstrating that those people who had no choice regarding entering an institution had a higher mortality rate after admission than those for whom other alternatives were available (although a causal relationship was not demonstrated) and that the way the relocation process is man-aged may influence mortality rates. In assessing the process of care, the question should be asked whether all of the possible choices for care were fully explored and presented to the client for consideration, selec-tion, or rejection.

Another essential component to consider is whether the client's social support system was identified and involved. Adequate social support may mitigate the health effects of some of the most disrupting events of later life (Minkler, 1985).

Because the case manager typically arranges for direct service delivery by other providers (ranging from chore and homemaker services, home health aides, in-home nursing services, durable equipment suppliers, to recommendations for physicians and nursing homes), another com-ponent in assessing the process of care is an evaluation of the service provided by the "subcontractors." If there is a perceived problem with quality, case managers must be empowered to discuss it with the "subcontractor" and find alternative referral resources if the quality problem is an unresolvable situation.

RELEVANCE OF HOSPICE CONCEPTS OF CARE IN CASE MANAGEMENT

There is only one "final placement," and it is neither the home or the nursing home. It is when the body is lowered into the grave. If the "final placement" is the grave, then the "penultimate placement" is increasingly the hospice. Families and clients enrolling in hospice care generally have very favorable things to say about their experiences with hospice, despite the fact that the final outcome is death. The main goal in hospice care is that of quality, as opposed to duration, of remaining life. One intervention for improving quality of life in hospice care is symptom control. Two other equally important concepts in hospice care, however, are enhancing the client's sense of control over the situation and augmenting the effectiveness of the social support network.

Individuals arriving at hospice have been given terminal prognoses, such that there is some degree of certainty or agreement that they are not likely to live beyond six months or so, regardless of professional interventions. There is generally less certainty about the anticipated time of death with the clients in a general geriatric case-management service. Yet, case managers would do well to consider, and perhaps adopt, a hospicelike philosophy in their approach to the frail elderly client, i.e., instead of asking, "How can this person live as long as possible in the lowest risk situation at any personal cost or burden?" the critical question is rather, "How can I help this person live most fully during the days she has remaining?" To answer this question, the case manager would need to know the values, preferences, and wishes of the client as well as the human relational context of family and friends that creates meaning for the individual. If the individual client were no longer able to express her values, preferences, and wishes, the case manager must rely on the family and friends to provide the information and guidance.

As long as the focus is kept on the quality of life as perceived by the client instead of the duration of days, the case manager will likely be guided into fewer truly bad outcomes. In most of medicine, and perhaps in most of case management as well, death is considered de facto a bad outcome. The skilled case manager, however, will discover for individual clients whether potential outcomes exist that are deemed worse than death, will explore why that is the case, and will be guided by that knowledge.

LANGUAGE AND HIDDEN ASSUMPTIONS

One perhaps not so hidden assumption in these case descriptions is found in the title of this section. That is the concept of "placement." This term is used commonly when referring to creating hospital discharge "dispositions" for old and frail people, that is, will the person be subjected to "nursing home placement." Objects are placed, such as placing an item on a shelf. When one considers placing a living being on a shelf (e.g., a cat), the placement is certainly not permanent or final because the living being will move itself. As part of the objectification of the cognitively or physically impaired, our language contains unspoken clues about our perceptions. If the person no longer retains the capability to execute her desires, she is less than human; she is an object needing a "disposition" (to be disposed of), needing "placement" (to be placed as though inanimate). Perhaps the only way for an elderly person to leave a situation in which she has been involuntarily "placed" is to exert her will to sever the psychic thread that holds an old body and soul together.

In arriving at recommendations concerning optimal or appropriate locations for clients to live, case managers would do well to avoid the language of objectification. Consciously speaking of "nursing home admission" instead of "nursing home placement" may help keep case managers cognizant of the distinction between a being versus an object. Similarly, case managers might ask themselves, "Why is this frail elderly person still living? What keeps this person connected to this earthly existence?" It is typically connections to people, animals, places, anticipation of events in the future, or unresolved issues of the past. Recognition of impaired individuals as truly human, and appropriate recognition and valuation of their earthly connectedness will guide the case manager into fewer bad outcomes.

CASE MANAGER AS SALESPERSON

When a case manager assesses a situation and reaches a professional opinion about what would in her estimation be best for the client, she may then find herself in the awkward position of having to sell the opinion to the client and the family. She may find herself truly believing in the product she is selling, or she may feel like the used car salesman who has the potential for pushing a real lemon. In the scenarios presented, the clients are subjected to "persuasion," to "giving in," to "having everyone gang up on them," to "the authority of the physician." Although there are circumstances in which it may be appropriate for the case manager to sell a particular viewpoint, when resistance is encountered the case manager must make a careful reassessment of her role. Who is she representing? Is anyone serving as advocate for the opinion of the client? How do the values, preferences, and wishes of the client mesh with the plan being sold? If they are in conflict, what considerations may override the wishes of the client? Is the client capable of making her own decisions in this matter? If the case manager becomes too zealous a salesperson for a particular plan of care that is in conflict with the client's values, preferences, and wishes, the potential for bad outcomes increases.

WHY NURSING HOME ADMISSIONS ARE CONSIDERED BAD OUTCOMES

An old woman living in a San Francisco nursing home once commented to Imogene Cunningham (1977), "When you come here nobody knows where you are." In this statement she captured the essence of one reason why nursing homes are considered bad outcomes. They are typically divorced from the community. When a person enters a nursing home, she may lose the connectedness to her family, friends, church, pets, familiar surroundings and furnishings, and other elements that give her life meaning. Her case manager and physician may no longer be able to work with her in the nursing home, which may represent the severing of long-time relationships. If the boundaries of the nursing home were more fluid with respect to the community and pre-established social support networks, nursing homes would perhaps not be considered categorically bad.

Instead of choosing the nursing home as one possibility from a menu of quality options, the nursing home is usually considered the default option, when all other aspects of caregiving systems have failed. It is feared worse than death for many older people because of the associated fear of abandonment, loss of autonomy, and demise in what is perceived to be an unsupportive, understaffed, underskilled setting. While the people entering nursing homes as residents often do so because they have no other options, the people working in nursing homes likewise are often there because other options do not exist for them in the workforce. When default option residents who don't want to be there are cared for by default option employees who similarly would rather be elsewhere, it is difficult to expect the chemistry of a positive environment.

Entering a nursing home should not have to be necessarily a bad outcome. In our present day collective psyche, however, it is. No one wants to live in an institution. As long as nursing homes are perceived to be rigid and regimented institutions, they will be considered bad outcomes for most people.

The nursing home of the future may present to a client a constellation of benefits and options within a setting that is more accurately characterized as a congregate living center than an institution. Although great strides have been made in improving the quality of care delivered in our nation's nursing homes, the day remains in the future when entering a nursing home will be a highly valued option for its strong sense of community, the individualized and attentive care given there, the sense of peace for the client and family arising from a secure and comfortable environment, and the knowledge that the nursing home is an integrated and integral part of the community. Only when nursing homes become places through which (instead of within which) people can live their remaining days fully will they lose their current cultural connotations as in and of themselves bad outcomes.

REFERENCES

Cunningham, I. (1977). *After ninety*. Seattle, WA: University of Washington Press.

Kasl, S. V. (1972). Physical and mental health effects of involuntary relocation and institutionalization on the elderly—a review. *American Journal of Public Health, 62*, 377-384.

Minkler, M. (1985). Social support and health of the elderly. In S. Cohen & S. L. Syme (Eds.), *Social support and health*. New York: Academic Press.

Rodin, J. (1986). Aging and health: Effects of the sense of control. *Science, 233*, 1271–1276.

Rowe, J. W. & Kahn, R. L. (1987). Human aging: Usual and successful. *Science, 237*, 143–149.

VIEW FROM THE FIELD

Perspective From Oregon

■

Susan Dietsche

The following guidelines should be used in shaping the case manager's responsibilities:

1. Clients need to determine the settings of their care. The earlier that a client considers the choices the better. The decision also needs to be made on *good* information regarding "needs" and resources available for meeting needs, that is, what are Miss E and her sister able to manage or tolerate to remain at home? Does the sister need some respite? How are the "4 hours" of help used? Are there other family members or friends to provide support to the sister? Is housekeeping and "eating well" important? What was the life-style before deterioration? If Miss E "agrees" to go to a nursing home, what kind of preparation and support does she need?

2. Case-management programs *must* maximize the type of options available for care settings. From the limited information available, it appears that the two sisters might be willing to move to an apartment-like setting that preserves the independence of home and privacy, and yet provides access to the necessary social and medical support required by *both* sisters. In Oregon, assisted living or even Adult Foster Care might meet that requirement.

3. Several factors should be taken into account in determining placement. The most important may be the ability or willingness of the client to give up *autonomy* (to whatever degree) to achieve *comfort* or "care" (whatever the degree). This is a preference that may have been reflected in life-style over many years, or may be determined by asking.
   The most difficult factor to plan around is the effect of the decisions on others, including the public's health, effects of sanitary threats, bizarre behavior, or self-neglect. But even this factor has to be addressed in a way that maximizes the person's autonomy at least to the degree that one assesses the client has a strong preference for autonomy.

4. The effect of bad outcomes in the past is part of the experience and knowledge of the case manager. Death is not a bad outcome if

the client has had some influence on the environment in which it occurs. In fact, death is inevitable. The "bad" part of the outcome is if the client missed the chance to have some control over the way in which the event occurred.

5. Nursing home admissions are not categorically bad, just like hospital admissions or outpatient treatment by physicians are not bad. What is categorically bad is the inability to have some say or control over the event or not to have had the opportunity to plan in advance on how to meet long-term care needs. A person may choose to convalesce in a medical setting (i.e., nursing home). Rehabilitative services, if extensive, may be available only in a nursing home, and 24-hour nursing care, if not available from a friend or family, may be provided most economically in a nursing home. If a person requires comfort and care on a 24-hour basis and cannot afford alternatives, the nursing home would be most appropriate.

EDITORS' QUESTIONS FOR FURTHER DISCUSSION

∎

1. To what extent should clients determine the settings of their care? Are family concerns relevant?
2. To what degree should case-management programs maximize the type of options available for care settings?
3. What factors are reasonable to consider in determining placement?
4. How should previous bad outcomes in other cases be considered?
5. Should case managers judge nursing home admissions as categorically bad?
6. Is the language of "placement" inherently dehumanizing? What terms could be substituted?

Chapter 9

SECRETS: Confidentiality and Disclosure in Case Management

CASE

∎

The case-management agency in county X is in an uproar because of confidentiality issues. They just seem too complicated to get right and rules to cover these situations might help. Of course, the agency has a release form that must be signed before information about the client is disclosed. It says that no information will be shared beyond the case-management team without specific consent from the client except for the minimal information that care providers who come to the home will need to give the right care. This should work but it doesn't.

The current uproar is because last week one of the town councilwomen called to ask about a client's well-being and Miss Smith, the case manager, said she couldn't disclose any information. The particular client is a bit eccentric, and tends not to elicit much sympathy in the community, but the case manager thinks the principle would be the same regardless of who the client is or what the inquirer wants to do with the information. But by the end of the day, there was a staff meeting, and case managers were instructed that when people in the community call with an interest in helping the client, case managers should cooperate and tell them what they want to know. The case managers are angry about that, but the supervisor pointed out that there will be no program at all if the community leaders are alienated.

Moreover, if case managers are close-mouthed, sometimes community leaders think that the agency isn't doing its job right when actually the clients have refused help for various reasons. Surely, the supervisor argues, it is okay to explain circumstances like this. Do the case managers want to see the whole program get a bad reputation or be closed down? Don't citizens have a legitimate interest in understanding what the case managers do?

This week's crisis is just the tip of the confidentiality iceberg. Problems regularly arise regarding the home care providers and other agencies with which the case manager works. For example, case managers often want to explain some things to home care providers so that they will know what to expect and give better care, but they are supposed to be cautious in this regard. They aren't supposed to mention mental health problems of the client, for example. In one case, Miss Smith felt really guilty because she knew that the client's 55-year-old son had served time for sexual assault and couldn't mention it to the agency that was contracted to provide care. Instead she suggested the agency send a male personal care aide but did not explain why.

And confidentiality must even apply to disclosures to family members. They sure don't understand your position when you refuse to tell them what their mother or father has said or thinks. Some case managers say that information works both ways—if you want information from the family member, you have to give a little, too. Case managers walk a thin line. Once one of the case managers called a client's daughter and mentioned that her mother seemed to be having trouble paying her bills, and the client called her up in outrage: "You told my daughter. . . ." Well, what should she have done? The case managers are *supposed* to get families involved in care. Furthermore, family members also tell the case managers things and expect their own confidentiality to be observed. Not infrequently both family and doctor are keeping the patient's diagnosis a secret. Sometimes the family wants to keep their intent to arrange a nursing home a secret from the client or other relatives. What does the case manager do here?

Ms. Private, a case manager from the branch office in a small rural town pointed out that, at least for her, confidentiality is really a myth. Everyone knows everyone else, and all their relatives, and their dogs and cats. Everyone knows what work the case manager does, and when she comes to visit someone in the senior apartment building everyone else notices. This rural case manager thinks the best solution here is to avoid learning things. She suggests that the standardized assessment is much too intrusive, that they ask about things that are none of their business, that sometimes it is just curiosity that is served rather than need to know. She also thinks that if clients really understood what happens with information, they wouldn't tell one third of what they do. Others disagree completely with this case manager and argue that responsible case management must be based on a complete multidimensional assessment and that case managers, indeed, need to know the information they ask.

Even the mandated reports give some case managers a problem. One indicated that a client confided physical abuse (which must be reported) to the case manager, but then wept and pleaded with her not to tell anyone. The client had not known beforehand that the case manager would be obliged to call authorities. The client said she was an adult, that she understood her son's problems, and that if she had wanted to call authorities she could have done it herself. She felt that she was being discriminated against because she was old. Although the case manager resisted the impulse to keep quiet and made the report, she wondered if it really was so important for her to report the suspected abuse.

COMMENTARIES

Uses and Abuses of Confidentiality

■

Rosalie A. Kane

People want to be understood and admired. They like to be treated as individuals, and some even like to hear their words quoted and taken seriously. Yet people also dread being inaccurately characterized, becoming the subject of idle conversation, or having intimate information indiscriminately disclosed. The more clients tell their case managers, the more likely they will be to experience both the positive and negative consequences of having their business and their feelings known and understood. The hodge-podge of situations involving confidentiality and disclosure and case management in the agency depicted in this case cry out for an organizing rubric to help determine what a case manager should ask and of whom, and what a case manager should tell and to whom. This comment begins with the issues of confidentiality in the context of case management, from which follows approaches to the problems posed in the case.

BASIS FOR RESPECTING CONFIDENTIALITY

Controlling the flow of information about oneself and the communication of one's ideas and feelings seems to be a natural desire. This prerogative is generally recognized for all but the most public of figures, and carries with it the utilitarian advantage of perceived and actual control in one's environment. Showing how far this principle has been taken in American life, as I write this comment, a young man has just been awarded substantial monetary and punitive damages from a high school district because his grades were disclosed at a school board meeting.

Respect for the privacy of others has been elevated to a moral duty (though not an absolute duty) in various ethical formulations. The biblical tradition holds that Moses' sister Miriam was punished with leprosy for the sin of gossiping. Generations of mothers have taught their children that "if you can't say anything nice, say nothing at all," thus condoning testimonials while proscribing critical disclosures. Philosophers refer to the principle of respect for the autonomy of persons as the grounding for the duty to treat confidentially personal information about others (whether the information is observed, learned serendipitously, or openly disclosed). Not only does autonomy entail freedom to determine how information about oneself is used, but some degree of privacy seems to be a prerequisite for autonomous decision-making and action (Beauchamps & Childress, pp. 329–340; Walters, 1991).

Building on this general thinking (and adding an element of self-interest, discussed later) professionals tend to have inserted "confidentiality clauses" in their codes of ethics, whether these are recognized fully in law (e.g., as is true for attorneys and clergy), recognized substantially (as is true for physicians, who are expected to treat information confidentially, but to disclose any information vital to the public's health), or unrecognized and ambiguous under the law (as is true for social workers, who have responsibilities to the public as well as their clients, and who also work with families and communities and are, thus, often unclear about whom confidentiality is owed). Legal protection of communication notwithstanding, however, professionals argue that confidentiality is important both because privacy is an absolute value based on the principle of autonomy, and because more good than harm will occur if professionals who depend on disclosures from clientele or other sources encourage candor through promises of confidentiality than if professionals were not bound by this promise. Of course, once a promise or implied contract is involved, further ethical demands are placed on the person entering into the agreement, again based on the principle of respect for the autonomy of persons and the duty to follow through with promises.

CASE MANAGEMENT CONTEXT

Case managers thrive on information. They seek it to enhance their understanding of their client's situation, and they use it to plan the care. A comprehensive assessment is at the heart of the case management process, and the ability to synthesize and use information is a hallmark of a skilled case manager (Applebaum & Austin, 1990; Kane, 1990).

The routine initial assessment takes more than an hour to perform. It includes a series of structured questions about the client's or perspective client's past and present. The assessment is typically done in the client's own home, where the case manager is privy to details that an office setting would leave concealed. Areas usually part of the formal assessment battery include physical health, including checklists of illnesses, symptoms, recent use of care, and medications; functional abilities including self-care abilities (such as dressing, bathing, eating, getting in and out of bed, and using the toilet) and independent living skills (such as cooking, cleaning, laundry, transporting oneself, using money, and communicating orally and in writing); emotional states (depression, anxiety, psychiatric history and current symptoms, alcohol use); cognitive abilities (usually measured by a series of questions testing recent and remote memory, judgments, and arithmetic skills); social functioning including a summary of the relationships among family and friends and the amount of help received); adequacy of the living environment; and patterns of help currently received from all paid and unpaid sources. Income amounts and sources are, of course, part of the assessment, and this information may be necessary to establish program eligibility (Kane & Kane, 1981).

Such an assessment leaves few personal stones unturned. During the assessment, clients are expected to disclose problems, weaknesses, and feelings of an intimate nature, including seldom-discussed matters of urinary accidents and toileting needs. They are expected to discuss the kind of help they receive or want to receive from relatives. The case manager's question may be a routine item about how often the client sees her daughter, but the truthful answer may entail an embarrassing disclosure for a client who feels ill used or neglected by that daughter or, conversely, who harbors a wish to see less of that daughter.

The assessment is written down and becomes part of a record. Increasingly, parts of such records are computerized. The case manager continues to monitor the case once the initial plan is in effect, collecting additional information and updates. Every so often the case manager does a formal reassessment. The quality of a case manager's performance is judged, in part, by the skill and thoroughness of the assessment, and the extent to which the plan is tailored to fit the client as revealed by the assessment.

The information the case manager learns and the feelings the case manager elicits are, by definition, personal. Ms. Private's uneasiness with the intrusiveness of the assessments and her preference not to ask and not to know are natural reactions. They are particularly likely reactions if the case manager has no general professional training or specific training in assessment to overcome embarrassment and to respond appropriately to the feelings her questions elicit.

But, although Ms. Private would prefer that the assessment be minimized, arguably case managers show greater disrespect for older persons when they form judgments about their capabilities and well-being without asking them than when case managers go ahead and pose the personal questions. Indeed we have argued in another context that the assessment should be *extended* to inquire systematically about the values and preferences of the clients. With a grant from the Retirement Research Foundation, we are developing and testing just such an approach. Further, case managers have observed that elderly clients are often willing and even sometimes relieved to talk about themselves, their lives, and their problems. Indeed, case managers may have more difficulty limiting their time with garrulous clients than teasing information from taciturn ones.

To sort out the many questions about confidentiality in County X's case management program, we need to consider some basic questions: (a) What does the case manager need to know to do the job, and why? (b) What should become part of the permanent record? (c) What understandings should exist between case manager and client about the reason the information is being sought, the way it will be used, and the client's rights to refuse to answer? (d) Under what circumstances should information be shared?

Regarding the first question, the case manager needs some information to establish eligibility for services and to set priorities among the client's need and those of others as a basis for a care plan that is adequate for the particular client and equitable to all clients (Kane, 1992). Considerable additional information is needed to assess the issues in a case, determine whether rehabilitation with the goal of improved functioning is feasible, and developing an individualized plan. Furthermore, the relationship of trust and understanding between case manager and client will be enhanced by an exchange that goes beyond the superficial. The trust thus engendered enhances the likelihood that the client will keep the case manager informed as the case progresses and turn to the case manager at times of crisis.

Regarding the second question, every detail need not be incorporated into a formal record. The case manager can keep some elaborations out of the record. But, to document eligibility to ensure continuity of service, and to avoid duplicative assessments on the part of each provider, much of the information needs to be written down. However, clearer understandings are needed about the extent to which personal identifications should be incorporated into higher levels of aggregation. For example, for the state's planning purposes, it is unnecessary to have individual identifiers, but to track clients' well-being over time, longitudinal data must be kept somewhere.

Regarding the third question, the client needs to know why the questions are being asked and how the information will be used. County X had a routine release form that the client signed indicating the parameters under which information would be disclosed—namely, that only the case management team would share the assessment except for minimal information that would be provided to persons working in the home. We are given few details about the consent process. The consent request is hardly informative unless the client knows who is considered part of the case-management team, and what it means to disclose information to providers. For example, they should know whether information would be disclosed to the provider agency or the paraprofessional home care worker or both, and whether such information would be limited to disclosure of the client's physical needs. Among the items that should be explained when applicable are the following: that the assessment is used to determine services that the client may be eligible for and that might be helpful; that the case manager's role involves working with clients so that they can together achieve an understanding of the problems and the possibilities for solving them; that when possible the case manager attempts to incorporate family help into the care plan, and, therefore, will be asking questions of and about family members; and that although the client need not answer all the questions, the case manager may be unable to establish eligibility for service unless responses are forthcoming to various key questions. In a publicly funded program, the client's freedom to decline to answer some questions is contingent on being willing to forego the possible benefits. The case manager should clarify, however, *which* questions are necessary to establish the eligibility (usually questions about income and about functional disabilities), and which ones are optional but useful to allow the case manager to understand the client and help him or her better. Similarly, if family members are "assessed" as part of the comprehensive assessment, they must be informed about the extent to which their disclosures are confidential and whether they will be shared with the client.

The fourth question—under what circumstances will the information about the client be shared?—comes to the heart of the dilemmas that have arisen in our case. The case involved possible sharing of information with family members, direct care providers to whom referrals have been made (some of whom are under contract with the case management agency), and the general public. It involves different types of disclosures: those that come from answering direct questions, those initiated by the case manager, and those that arise from the case manager being observed (especially in rural communities). Handling information and behaving discreetly will minimize the latter type of disclosure and is particularly important in small communities where the web of social and work-related relationships is tight. The case manager might well think differently about disclosures that involve answering questions and those that involve imparting information at their own initiative. With the former, the case manager often can exercise the option of discussing the request with the client and determining if the client would prefer to remain private, and whether he or she would welcome direct questions from the relative, neighbor, or agency that inquired or prefer that the case manager serve as an intermediary.

Reasons for the disclosures by case managers also vary and include the case manager wants to eliminate misunderstandings and increase understanding about the client on the part of family, other professionals, or care providers; the case manager wants to prepare providers to help the client more effectively; the case manager wants to warn providers about possible risks and dangers to them in the caregiving situation; the case manager wants to satisfy curiosity, defuse criticism, or justify the actions of the case management agency. Some reasons for disclosures seem more valid than others. The most compelling reason to disclose information about the client is to protect others from a clear danger, followed by the beneficent motivation to improve the care the client receives.

Disclosures to providers would be largely unnecessary if each agency were expected to conduct its own detailed assessment of the client's needs, but arguably such duplicative assessments are burdensome for clients. They are also expensive to perform and thus undercut resources available for direct service.

How will the client be informed about particular disclosures, and what disclosures can the client veto? The blanket permission to disclose a wide range of information as the case manager sees fit (agency X's release form) seems an unjustifiable policy from an ethical standpoint. In most instances, the case manager should request the client's permission before discussing his or her case. In instances in which the case manager has no discretion but must make disclosures, the client should be informed, in advance, if possible, about what will be disclosed and why. If advance disclosure is impossible, the client should be informed as soon as possible about what has been disclosed and why. There will be little argument about mandatory referrals to police or protective authorities in situations in which the client is being harmed or is harming someone else. Case managers are more likely to be conflicted about whether they should disclose information in instances in which judgments of client or societal risk are involved (e.g., suicide risk or self-neglect) or in instances in which they sympathize with a client's subversion of a rule (e.g., a client's failure to report assets fully or a client's violation of a technical eligibility requirement).

Regarding discretionary disclosures, if the case manager can explain that the client will get better service if the case is explained to providers, clients will usually agree to such information sharing. Few would object if the home care worker were briefed on the client's history of heart disease and what to do in an emergency, or if the home care worker were told about a disabled person's request that her son not be admitted to the house because of previous theft and harassment. If clients do object, I argue the program should not share information until they convince the client that such disclosure is desirable. Procedures could be devised to clarify the case manager's intentions, promote accuracy, and reassure clients. Particularly worth exploring and testing is a process wherein the case managers make a brief (e.g., one-page) summary of salient information that would be shared with providers and get prior approval from the client for its use. As far as I know, no case-management organization has developed such approaches.

WHO IS THE CLIENT?

The issue of disclosures among family members is complicated by ambiguity about who the client is. If the case manager (in true social work tradition) considers the family to be the client, an open communication within the client system is suggested. However the phrase "family-as-client" needs specification: Does this mean the marital pair, the household, or the entire extended family? Although families are usually benign and supportive, sometimes family interests are at odds with those of clients and occasionally families are downright malevolent. If the client is incompetent, a family member is typically the client's official agent and must then be considered as the client, but the issue of how that agent is viewed vis-à-vis other family members still remains. Certainly there is much room for development of theory in this arena, but my predisposition would be not to assume that a competent adult client or a proxy for an incompetent client automatically agrees to share information with all or even any family members. Instead I would ask the client (or proxy) about such information sharing and take my cue from there. If the client wishes not to disclose information routinely to family members, say, a spouse or a daughter, this would need to be respected, and the rules for disclosures already discussed would apply. That is, at times, because of extreme risks to the family member or the client or others in the community, the case manager may have to tell the family member something and inform the client about what he or she will tell or (if after the fact) has told. At other times, the case manager will have a beneficent motivation for wanting to disclose to family members, but will be obligated to convince the client and get permission before going ahead. And sometimes the client will indicate that he or she has no secrets from some subset of his or her family, and the case manager can then communicate with the family group openly.

CONFIDENTIALITY AS A SHIELD FOR THE CASE MANAGER

So far we have discussed confidentiality as something that is preserved for the sake of the autonomy, dignity, and well-being of the client. But to be complete, another motivation for confidentiality must be aired. Sometimes professionals and organizations use the cloak of confidentiality to prevent scrutiny of their behavior and accountability for their actions, an issue that has been discussed in reference to secrecy in the doctor-patient relationship (Bok, 1983). Under the rubric of protecting client confidentiality, agencies can avoid scrutiny on things gone wrong. Yet, city and county officials and the taxpayer deserve to have some questions answered about an agency that it has entrusted to perform an important social function. Sometimes family members who believe their relative has been ill served also deserve to have their questions answered. Mechanisms for answering questions while preserving truly confidential information must be developed, and mechanisms for full-scale inquiries (in which some client information is disclosed) may also be needed.

RETURN TO CASE

Let's now turn to our case and see how our analysis of the issues concerning confidentiality and disclosure would suggest we should resolve the specific questions in the case. Let's take them in the order they occur in the narrative.

The town councilwoman should not have received specific information about Miss Smith's client. There seemed to be no need to know about this particular townsperson's business. The supervisor was wrong to capitulate to public clamor and fail to support his case manager. However, the councilwoman's questions should be handled with tact and responsiveness in terms of explaining how the agency functions in general. If the councilwoman were embarking on a legitimate inquiry because of a concern about the agency's practices, however, it would be necessary for the agency to find a way to offer relevant facts without jeopardizing client privacy. The agency cannot assume there is no legitimate public interest in its behavior.

Regarding general explanations to home care providers and other agencies, the case managers can explain the client's situation and functional need with the client's permission and within parameters already discussed with the client. The case manager should consider preparing a written statement for the client's review so that clients will know how their case is discussed, but, in any event, the case manager should indicate to the client the extent and substance of the planned disclosures to providers. If the agency routinely sends a complete copy of the assessment to the provider agencies, the client must know this practice occurs, know what is written down and what is verbally communicated, and give consent beforehand to the process. If the client refuses to have some or all information disclosed, the case manager should generally respect that request. The mental health history of the client is usually irrelevant to the provider. If the case manager thinks it is relevant, he or she needs to make that case convincingly enough to the client to get permission. If actual or imminent serious harm to the client or others is at stake, the obligation to secrecy does not hold. Regarding the potential danger of assault of a home care worker by a clients' family, for example, the case manager should inform the provider agency about any risks he or she thinks are substantial. Oblique suggestions that the agency should send a male worker to this home are a failure of the case manager's obligation because they do not constitute true communication. Workers go alone into people's homes and are vulnerable. The case manager needs to tell the home care agency what the issues are, and let the client know (preferably in advance but at least after the fact) what was communicated. Of course, if the case manager judges that the situation for a home worker is enormously risky (e.g., the client has a gun and indicates that he will kill anyone who comes to clean the house), there will be no need for disclosure to a home care agency, because no referral can be responsibly made. Probably, the case manager will need to inform other authorities about this danger.

The questions about what family members should be told can be teased out based on the previous discussion. Unless the case manager has been given blanket permission by the client, he or she must refuse to explain to relatives what the client thinks or to offer opinions about the client's functioning. If relatives fail to understand that position, as the worker in this case thinks is likely, perhaps the case manager has not explained her role effectively. The case manager should *not* have telephoned a client's daughter to warn her that her mother was having trouble paying the bills. Family members and physicians should *not* keep the patient's diagnosis a secret, and indeed family members should not get a preview of the diagnosis in advance of the client except in emergency situations (e.g., permission for surgery is needed for an unconscious patient). The case manager should *never* collude with family by concealing an intent to arrange a nursing home admission from the person to be admitted. This unfortunate practice, which occurs more than one would expect, is unethical on the part of all concerned—family members and professionals.

Ms. Private has exaggerated the problem of keeping information confidential. She hopes that by throwing up her hands in despair and saying that confidentiality is a myth in a rural community, she is absolved of the need to do full assessment and to act with discretion. Her view that it is better not to know things or inquire too deeply is simplistic. She is right that idle curiosity is a poor motivation for seeking information. But a certain amount of interest and curiosity about our fellow human beings (tinged with empathy and goodwill) is what makes good case managers as well as good therapists, social workers, novelists, and even good friends. A case manager who cares too little to wonder about the reason for a client's disabilities, fears, hopes, and plans is unlikely to engender confidence or to arrive at an individualized and sensitive care plan. The case manager should be aware that comprehensive assessment of another human being is an act of hubris, and mindful that a person cannot be encapsulated by a series of scores and answers to questions. But in humility and modesty, the case manager should attempt to learn about the client in depth and then respect that information in the ways we have discussed.

About the mandated report of abuse, the case manager is stuck. She must report it. If she thinks that the definitions used in her state and the state-reporting requirements are in error, her obligation is to work toward policy change.

CONCLUSION

Confidentiality is not an absolute principle for case managers, but it is an important one considering the kinds of information case managers seek. I argue they should continue to seek such personal information, and that mutual examination of such information will permit an important trust to develop between client and case manager, and will allow the latter to understand the client enough to really help. However, clients should be told in advance what kinds of questions are being asked and why, what will be done with the information, whether they may decline to reply, and the consequences of such a refusal.

Moreover, case managers themselves should know why they collect information and how to use assessment data. It should not be equated with the mechanics of "paperwork." Case-management agencies should explore consent protocols and ways of transferring information that clarify the process for clients and respect their privacy maximally. Providers and family members should not receive information about a competent client without the client's consent, except when such disclosures avert actual or imminent serious harm. In such instances, when information is given without a client's prior consent, the client should be informed. If no emergency exists, the case manager may and should attempt to persuade a client that it is in his or her interest to allow information to be shared and why. And, finally, the case-management program must not hide behind a cloak of client confidentiality to avoid public accountably and criticism, or to side-step legitimate inquiries from concerned relatives of the client.

A decade after confidentality in medicine has been challenged as "a decrepit concept (Siegler, 1982), we cannot be naïve about the practical limits of confidentality for a role as diffuse, variable, and ill defined as case management. All the more reason, it seems to me, to work diligently toward a set of well-understood ground rules about privacy and disclosure, and develop procedures for responsible exchange of information. Haphazard and ad hoc solutions will undermine confidence in the case management enterprise.

REFERENCES

Applebaum, R., & Austin, C. (1990). *Long-term care case management*. New York: Springer.

Beauchamp, T. L., & Childress, J. F. (1989). *Principles of biomedical ethics* (3rd ed.). New York: Oxford University Press.

Bok, S. (1983). The limits of confidentiality. *The Hastings Center Report*, *13*, 24–31.

Kane, R. A. (1990). Instruments to assess functional status. In C. K. Cassell, D. E. Reisenberg, L. B. Sorensen, & J. R. Walsh (Eds.), *Geriatric medicine*. New York: Springer-Verlag.

Kane, R. A. (1992). Case management in long-term care: It can be ethical and efficacious. *Journal of Case Management, 1*, 76–81.

Kane, R. A., & Kane, R. L. (1981). *Assessing the elderly: A practical guide to measurement*. New York: Springer.

Sielger, M. (1982). Confidentiality in medicine—a decrepit concept. *The New England Journal of Medicine, 307*, 1518–1521.

Walters, L. (1991). The principle of medical confidentiality. In Mappes, T. A., & Zembaty, J. S. (Eds.). *Biomedical ethics*. New York: McGraw-Hill.

The Community Need to Know:
Comments on a Secrecy Case[1]

■

Amitai Etzioni

DEONTOLOGICAL CONSIDERATIONS

Some of the questions in the case before us should be examined not only from a utilitarian-consequentialist viewpoint but also from the viewpoint of binding moral duties or deontology, which takes intentions into account. For example, if one donates blood and the patient dies (without any benefit from the donation) from a sheer utilitarian-consequentialist viewpoint, no moral act occurred. From a deontological perspective, if the actor proceeded to live up to her or his moral obligations (rather than to incur favor or gain a tax credit), donating blood is a moral act, whatever the consequences. (One may combine both considerations, as when one donates blood and considers a patient who is more likely to benefit from the donation. Either way, including deontological considerations often leads to morally sounder judgments (Etzioni, 1988).

---

[1] The author benefited from editorial comments by Brad Wilcox.

In the case at hand, one criteria for judging various acts is what was the intention? Did the council member call to inquire about the well-being of the patient to help a police investigation into a crime committed by the patient, to help raise funds needed for the person's care, to gossip, or to arrange for an organ donation? It may be said that intentions are hard to judge. However, we can judge our own intentions: Do we respond to a request to divulge information to help the patient or to help ourself? Accordingly, it seems less objectionable if a case manager told the children of a nursing home patient that she has a hard time paying her bill because the manager was concerned that the patient might be transferred for nonpayment and, consequently, be traumatized, as opposed to revealing the information in the hope of garnering a favor from the nursing home owner. Second, although we all have difficulties in forming definitive judgments about the intentions of others, we can—especially when we know them and are familiar with the situation—come to reasonable judgment. Case managers have more latitude when their intentions are primarily aimed to help the patient rather than themselves.

VALUE OF PRIVACY

One of the questions raised by the case before us is this: May one violate the privacy of the patient and under what conditions, if any? I shall argue that (a) all rights should be treated as relative and not as absolute ones; (b) that all rights of a person are limited by the rights of others; (c) that rights ought to be balanced with concerns about the needs of the community; and (d) finally that the right to privacy does not rank particularly high among our values and should not be treated as some kind of trump value.

Our tendency in recent years has been to treat rights as absolute. Rights have been formulated as if they were unbounded claims due us by nature or justice or as "inevitable." But, as Loren Lomasky (1987) writes,

> There is ample reason to view with alarm a public discourse that increasingly ascends (descends?) to the level of rights-talk. Problems tractable if formulated in terms of contending interests or preferences become rigidified when transformed into disputes over basic rights. This unfortunate escalation of charge and countercharge can take on the appearance of inevitability. (pp. 7–8)

In effect, rights may appear to us as commanding unmitigated loyalty but are all subject to some limitations (Lomasky, 1987; Morgan, 1984). Even the much revered First Amendment, often treated as if it was absolute, is circumscribed by the well-known prohibition against shouting "fire" in a crowded theater. All other rights are similarly conditional. All acts should be weighed as they are affected by and affect a variety of moral considerations.

Because the individuals who constitute a society all have the same rights, the rights of every individual must be limited by the rights of others. My freedom is limited by everyone else's freedom. My right to extend my fist stops at your nose.

Beyond the rights of others there are the needs of the community, values we all share, such as the environment (above and beyond the environmental rights of specific actors). These needs set further limits on the rights of us all. It is surprising how often this consideration is ignored. The liberal tradition "has tended to make [human] rights absolute, with no possibility of coordinating them with one another or with other social goods [and] when everyone seeks entitlement, society becomes ungovernable" (Gelpi, 1989).

For instance, when human immunodeficiency virus (HIV) testing is discussed, it is often suggested (by the American Civil Liberties Union, among others) that one reason such testing is inappropriate is that because there is no known cure, testing cannot help the HIV carrier. It is useless information for him or her. Moreover, test results may stigmatize a carrier, or prevent him or her from obtaining health services, and keeping a job and insurance. This radically individualistic position ignores the fact carriers must be concerned about infecting others and the effects of spreading the plague on the community. If a person exhaled cyanide, surely we would expect him or her to provide society with knowledge of that condition, enabling us to take the condition into account. HIV, with its 80% or higher fatality rate, should not be treated differently. As this issue demonstrates, when we address social needs, rights need to be balanced by community considerations.

Finally, with respect to privacy, a key value in the case at hand, it should be noted that privacy is not one of the rights as much as mentioned in the constitution. It was "added on" to the Constitution by legal theorists, lawyers, and judges. And, the right to privacy clearly has a lesser standing than, say, the First Amendment. This is revealed when these two values clash, because privacy tends to yield. Moreover, as Mary Ann Glendon spells out in her brilliant book, the notion of the right to be left alone has eaten into caring and sharing, the foundation of neighborhoods and communities. We have gone too far. As Glendon (1991) writes, the philosophical ideal of self-sufficiency that we have thus democratized is a state to which few men, and even fewer women, can aspire. By making a radical version of individual autonomy normative, we inevitably imply that dependency is something to be avoided in oneself and disdained in others. (p. 141)

Most important, privacy is primarily—if not completely—a legal concept. When we talk about the right not to be snooped on, "the privacy of one's bedroom" and so on, we typically refer to the need to curb the government, not mainly or firstly, to curb neighborhoods and communities. Thus, the core principle—the right to be left alone—applies to the government (unless a compelling reason is given otherwise, say, probable cause that the person is a criminal), but this is not the basis of neighborly and community conduct.

Here the opposite might be said to prevail: We are each others' keepers, unless there is a special reason not to keep one another. Thus, we do keep tabs on one another, but in a social context this is viewed as caring, even if it entails some form of behavior that if carried out by the government would be considered objectionable. Neighbors frequently do look into each others' backyards and beyond, and complain to other neighbors when they do not cut their grass or otherwise offend the communities' values and norms. Indeed, some forms of benign gossip (as distinct from malicious), what sociologists call informal communications, are a basis of community processes. Without them, we would not know who is in grief, down on their luck, and so on—that is, who needs special consideration and support, through sensitive and informal community mechanisms.

That does not mean that even in the social setting "anything goes" or that there is no communitarian, as opposed to legal, privacy. We cannot tap the neighbor's phone (even if we listen to what they say to the mail person), and we cannot open their mail. In short, the moral community standards of privacy are much narrower and less powerful than even the legal ones, which are far from absolute or preeminent.

BEARING ON THE CASE

The case before us, like many others, is complex in that many factors are operative and hence multiple considerations apply. There cannot be, and one ought not to seek, some simple or even not so simple a rule that will "tell us what to do." At best, we can have a set of guidelines that sensitize us and we draw on to help us form judgments in specific situations. In the case at hand, it seems justified to "violate" the patient's privacy when one or more of the following factors prevail.

Gravity

We should violate privacy when not doing so would gravely endanger the community or the lives of others, for example, if the person plans to poison the water main of another person. Or, to take another example, if he or she carries a contagious disease that has serious health consequences for others, say hepatitis B. In this case, I would favor (a) a moral expectation that the person who is a carrier will inform those he or she might have infected (for treatment and to curb further contamination), and all others before sustaining contact that might transmit the disease occurs; (b) that those who do not conduct themselves in that way be open to civil liability; (c) that they be required to inform public authorities, especially health care personnel, they come in touch with and allow their blood to be tested; (d) that health personnel be required to report cases and trace contacts; (e) that penalties will be significantly increased on those who violate the privacy of carriers *for other reasons* or those who discriminate against carriers in jobs, housing, and insurance. All this does not hold when the problem is relatively minor (flu) or intermittent (genital herpes).

Capacity of the Person

The case does not tell us if the patient does or does not have full mental capacity. Our ideology tends to assume that everybody including mental patients who roam the streets, have full capacity. I would hold that few do and that most people have some demonstrated mental incapacity, especially when under stress. Hence, they are entitled to varying degrees of help in making decisions, and information about their needs may be exchanged.

True and Hidden Preferences

The simple model of personal behavior on which radical individualists rely is that persons know their preferences (or at least are the best judges of what these preferences are) and that their preferences are basically straightforward, unincumbered, and certainly not internally contradictory or ambiguous. This, however, as Freud has argued, is not the common situation (Etzioni, 1988). Hence, when, for instance, Mrs. X complains to the case manager about telling her children about her predicament, it is not immediately clear what her actual preference is.

In an article entitled "Permissible Paternalism: In Defense of the Nanny State" Robert Goodin argued that although we should not act against a person's explicit well-established preference (e.g., to preach Zen Buddhism to a devout Catholic on his death bed), when we discern that there is a basic preference and a manifest one, we may respond to the basic one. Thus, if a person smokes but attended several clinics trying to stop smoking and keeps complaining about her habit, we may assume that the person actually seeks to refrain from smoking. By helping them to do so, even when not directly asked, we are in line with their basic or underlying preferences, and this does not constitute paternalism. In the case at hand, if the patient did not complain too much about passing on information to the children, if she continued to provide information to the case manager that might be passed along later but was not otherwise essential to her treatment, it would seem reasonable to interpret the situation as one in which she actually wished the information be transmitted. But this was also a case in which the client wished to save face, hence, the complaint. Case managers should have considerable latitude in interpreting these mixed messages and acting on their best judgment of what the patient's real preference is, especially when they are acting in line with the general welfare of the patient rather than their own.

REFERENCES

Etzioni, A. (1988). *The moral dimension*. New York: The Free Press.

Gelpi, D. (Ed.). (1989). *Beyond individualism*. Notre Dame, IN: Notre Dame University Press.

Glendon, M. A. (1991). *Rights talk*. New York: The Free Press.

Goodin, R. (1991). Permissible paternalism. In defense of the nanny state. *The Responsive Community, Rights and Responsibility, 1*, 42–51.

Lomasky, L. E. (1987). *Persons, rights and the moral community*. New York: Oxford University Press.

Morgan, R. (1984). *Disabling America*. New York: Basic Books.

VIEW FROM THE FIELD

Perspective From Washington

■

Charles E. Reed

A practical perspective from an operational level is also known as "being in the trenches," and it is here that "ethics" rears its head over and over. For it is at the worker level that ethical issues are grappled with, mulled over, discarded, or resolved so that a case manager can internalize and incorporate these ideas of confidentiality and informed consent into practice.

In "Secrets," it appeared that the case manager had undergone a process that for her was meaningful and followed that agency's confidentiality rules. However, enter the elected official inquiring about the client's well-being and being refused information on that basis, and a collision between the client's right to confidentiality and perceived notions about public officials duties occurs. Here, accountability is valued higher than the confidentiality issue. Perhaps the way to help citizens understand what case managers do is to send one to the city council meeting to explain their work and dilemmas. There are ways to educate the community other than breaking confidentiality.

Case managers are charged with helping clients understand why some information must be shared with providers. In the case of the client's son with the sexual assault record, careful probing and planning with the client might have led to a situation in which the client would have agreed to reveal this information. (In fact, the client may not have felt comfortable with a male personal care aide, and this might have been ignored in the rush to protect a worker without evading confidentiality.) In this example, the individual's comfort level in discussing the son's record was a basis for planning or decision making.

Working with clients, their families, and health practitioners can be difficult at best—training in family or group work will give the case manager a foundation on how to gather and disseminate information, and to assess and support a functional family system. In this context, confidentiality issues can be addressed. In another situation, there was a family doctor who did not divulge a diagnosis of cancer to a patient and her husband. Nieces and nephews knew of the diagnosis; the case manager and the registered nurse from the home health agency did not know. The client was on a behavior modification program because of her extreme dependence on her husband. He was unable to rest or sleep as the client demanded his presence at all times. She was hospitalized and died within 3 days. The family and doctor felt they had done the "best thing" for the client and her husband. Whenever possible, the case manager must urge for straightforwardness and honesty among all involved persons. But it is necessary to recognize the moment when the client and their families make their own decisions based on their values and family system. At that point, it's OK to let go.

Rural case managers are in peculiar positions. Friends and neighbors do know a great deal about one another and are generally aware of the case managers' duties and responsibilities. They will know why a case manager is visiting their neighbor or relative, and may think they know the intricacies of the situation. However, in performing an assessment only the client, case manager, and the people designated by the client will be privy to the information. This case manager may be uncomfortable in gathering information that she perceives as being intrusive and in maintaining boundaries with others about divulging information. Shortening an assessment because one perceives intrusiveness in its entirety may eliminate information that is necessary both for the case manager and the client. For it is through this assessment process that needs are identified and, with client involvement, plans are developed. If case managers decide what is to be assessed, clients are being patronized and not allowed to exercise self-determination.

Mandated reporting is a difficult issue that most human service professionals have faced at some time in their career. In this situation, some rapport had been developed with the case manager, which enabled the client to tell the case manager about the abuse she was experiencing. The case manager, through awareness of the dynamics of abuse, can then provide support and understanding to the client. In this way, the case manager can help the client understand that she doesn't have to endure abuse to understand her son's problems. If the potential for serious harm exists, she must report the situation no matter what the confidentiality rules are.

What our work in case management comes down to is training, informing the community about our work, support, and discussion. Training for the case manager in various clinical areas, such as family work, the cycles of abuse and violence, ways to deal with the inquiries, and identification of confidentiality issues should be ongoing in an agency. Educating the community about case management services and the roles and duties of case managers can be done in various ways, limited only by the imagination. In addition, it is imperative that support from supervisors, management, and agency policies provide the environment in which case managers can discuss these hard issues both with their peers and their supervisors. Agencies should involve staff in formulating and implementing policies and provide a formal mechanism for discussion of these issues.

EDITORS' QUESTIONS FOR FURTHER DISCUSSION

■

1. How should we define the community of "caregivers" for case-management clients? How much do caregivers and helpers of different training and background need to know about clients? Does it make a difference if the caregiver is a professional? Does it make a difference if the caregiver is a neighbor?
2. How should one weigh the privacy of the client against the needs and desires of others to know?
3. What are the boundaries of confidentiality within families? Should case managers keep client's secrets from family members? Should they keep family member's secrets from clients?
4. Do case managers seek to learn too much? Should assessments be more minimal and less personal?
5. When would breaking confidentiality be justified?
6. What would be an ideal consent form for case managers to use in seeking information from clients? In asking permission to disclose information?

Chapter 10

BEND OR SNAP: The Case Manager and the Rules

CASE

■

Mrs. B is a woman in her early 90s who doctors say will not survive for more than 6 months. She has multiple ailments including inoperable cancer. She has a large extended family who want to help her but have multiple demands that limit their ability. All relatives are poor and most work. The program can make payments for relatives to give care if the family qualifies because of low income, which the B's do. Mrs. B and her family agree that the best family caregiver would be Mona, her 17-year-old granddaughter. Mona dropped out of school last year and is willing to take care of her grandmother for the wage the state permits.

Unfortunately, the program does not permit payment to family caregivers under age 18. This is explained to the B's. They decide that another grandchild, Andrea, age 23 will give the care. Several months later, the case manager makes a visit and finds that Mona is in charge. Andrea is working at a restaurant, but gives the payments to Mona. Everyone is satisfied with the arrangement, and the care seems good. Mrs. B is dying, and she has the caregiver she prefers. What should the case manager do in the short run? She knows that if she tells her supervisor, payments for this care will cease. The rule says you need to be 18. The case manager keeps her mouth shut.

This case manager has another case that troubles her even more. She feels pretty firmly that the rule about age is arbitrary and a 17-year-old can give adequate care in some circumstances. However, in the C case, Mrs. C has a live-in unrelated caregiver who is paid by the program. Mrs. C has come to need some medically related care, including regular injections, that according to the state regulations should be done by a nurse. But if a nurse were paid to come in twice a day, then the program could no longer afford the main caregiver who does all the personal care and housekeeping. The case manager really thinks that the paraprofessional caregiver can do the tasks. Plenty of family members do similar things for their relatives—and it's legal as long as they are relatives. So the case manager leaves it alone and hopes for the best. But she wonders, is she doing the right thing? Is this case the same or different from the B case?

COMMENTARIES

When Breaking May Be Keeping

∎

Mary B. Mahowald

Every case is different. That's a truism to which both cases I have agreed to examine are no exception, despite their common elements. The key question they both raise occurs often in bureaucratic systems such as government, social service, and health care institutions. It is the question of whether individuals have the right or responsibility to break rules to promote the welfare of clients.

Discussions of this question have occurred over many years in the literature on civil disobedience. There is an important difference, however, between the arguments that literature provides for breaking laws or rules and these cases. The difference is that civil disobedience is traditionally practiced for the sake of a group rather than an individual. Unless decisions in both cases are made in behalf of classes of persons whose interests are unjustly undermined by the rules, they are not justifiable under the rubric of traditional civil disobedience. Advocacy for a client is not equivalent to advocacy for a class or group. Nevertheless, the issue of civil disobedience provides a useful paradigm through which to examine the central question raised by the cases involving clients B and C. In what follows, therefore, I examine the traditional doctrine of civil disobedience and apply it to the cases described. Preliminarily, I consider different views of the relationship between law and morality because it is that relationship on which arguments about keeping and breaking rules depend.

GENERAL CONSIDERATIONS

A law is a rule of conduct laid down by an authority within the community to which the rule applies. Examples include city statutes, state, or federal laws. Thomas Aquinas defines law as an ordinance of reason for the common good promulgated by one who has responsibility for the community (Aquinas, 1945). A statute based on reason for the common good is necessarily just.

To say that laws must be just is not to settle the question of the relationship between law and morality. Consider the following ways of viewing that relationship:

1. Law and morality are the same.
2. Law and morality are distinct.
3. Law and morality may be at odds.
4. Law and morality are complementary.
5. Law and morality overlap.

Most of us know individuals or cases that illustrate each of these views. I think of the obstetrician who delivered our first child, for example, who said that he never had to make a decision that was not already determined within the context of his own medical expertise or the laws of the place where he worked. Law, for him, *was* morality. Or I think of the neurologist who was asked by medical students about the legal parameters of a complicated case, who replied with evident pride: "I never consider the law in making decisions for patients." Morality in medical practice, he claimed, had nothing to do with the law.

Both of the preceding positions are simplistic. Laws cannot capture the more demanding and extensive reach of moral judgments, nor should they. Neither does it make sense to say that laws are morally irrelevant, because they do have consequences that should be considered in decision making, and they do at times articulate moral consensus on particular issues. Most of us, therefore, support a position between one that identifies morality with legality and one that treats them as totally separate spheres. To the extent that law and morality reflect different but nonconflicting views, they are complementary; to the extent that they are the same they of course overlap. To the extent that a law is unjust or otherwise immoral, we may either deny it *is* the law or view it as incompatible with morality. On either account, civil disobedience is justifiable and may even be morally obligatory.

The term *civil disobedience* may be misleading because in fact the practice involves obedience to law that is just. As Martin Luther King, Jr. (1962), put it, civil disobedience begins with recognition that certain rules or statutes are unjust because they are inequitably applied to some members of the community. Such injustice can only be recognized in light of recognition of the "higher" law of justice, which by some accounts is contained within the "natural law" that is part of the eternal law of God. The "higher" law of justice may also be accessible through conscience or through rational analysis. Most practitioners of civil disobedience have insisted on a collaborative effort to determine whether laws are in fact unjust. Only when injustice has been clearly established is civil disobedience justified as a means of rectifying the situation.

There are, of course, some familiar and well-respected historical examples of civil disobedients. In addition to King, Henry David Thoreau (1968) and Mahatma Gandhi (1961) come to mind, each exemplifying the fact that those who practice civil disobedience must accept the legal consequences of their actions. Socrates accepted the ultimate in legal penalties, capital punishment, when he was convicted of "crimes" of impiety and corruption of the youth of Athens (Plato, 1956). Faith in the capacity of a government to change its laws, and willingness to accept the consequences of challenging them, are prerequisites for the proper practice of civil disobedience. The illegal action undertaken by practitioners of civil disobedience is a sign intended to provoke those responsible for the law to recognize its injustice, so that they will voluntarily change it. Civil disobedience thus targets the conscience of lawmakers, assuming the ultimate persuasive strength of moral truth.

Traditionally, civil disobedience is also associated with nonviolence. While experiencing violence personally, even to the point of death, Gandhi and King remained unwilling to inflict violence on others. Those who joined them in their commitment to change unjust laws through civil disobedience were required to observe a similar commitment and to prepare themselves to withstand violence without returning it.

Those who reject civil disobedience as a moral mechanism for changing the law may not realize that it is based on respect for law and confidence that the legal system is capable of reforming itself. Although Socrates, Gandhi, and King might have avoided the legal penalties of their actions, they indicated their respect for the legal systems that governed their communities by choosing not to do so. Once confidence in the legal system is lost, as happened in some communities following the assassination of Martin Luther King, Jr., civil disobedience is no longer possible, and violent means of overcoming injustice may be undertaken (Malcolm X, 1966).

Clearly, most people who break laws are not practitioners of civil disobedience. Even the followers of Socrates, Gandhi, and King do not necessarily practice the rigorous demands of civil disobedience as historically presented. If breaking rules in cases such as those of clients B and C is to be morally justified, however, a rigorously understood concept of civil disobedience provides a solid and convincing rationale. Moreover, that same doctrine may be used to support the claim that breaking immoral laws is not only permissible but morally obligatory in some cases.

SPECIFIC CONSIDERATIONS

Some of the rules that appear to restrict the case manager in the cases described are consistent with laws that bind others in the community as well. The law excluding nonfamily members who are not clinicians from giving injections is an example of such consistency. A program rule that denies payment to a 17-year-old family caregiver probably also reflects state law even if it applies only to one program and has been developed by agency personnel rather than by legislators. Such rules simultaneously represent prima facie obligations for the case manager. Liability is probably only incurred by violation of rules that are formally laws. The case manager should be concerned about the liability incurred by permitting illegal provision of injections by an unrelated caregiver. Her concern illustrates the respect for law that is a component of civil disobedience. Ordinarily, the greater the authority of the law, the greater the burden of observing it and of ascertaining its injustice before civil disobedience is undertaken. Institutional rules are thus subject to city statutes, which are subject to state laws, which are subject to federal laws, which, in turn, are subject to the U.S. Constitution. The law preempting provision of injections by nonrelatives who are not clinicians would thus require a more compelling rationale for its violation than the program rule precluding Mona's acting as caregiver for her grandmother.

Respect for laws or rules involves acknowledgment of one's own nearsightedness or fallibility, and appreciation for the fact that laws are (or ought to be) developed collaboratively and rationally for the good of the community. But because human beings are fallible collectively as well as individually, human laws are not absolute. In other words, rules are means rather than ends. If they obstruct rather than facilitate the achievement of their (good) ends, they are no longer justifiable means. At that point, the moral thing to do is to attempt to change the laws. Whether one is morally obliged to observe the laws while involved in this attempt depends on whether the harm of obeying is greater than that of disobeying. Civil disobedience is an effort to change unjust laws, and not simply an act intended to benefit a single individual.

The circumstances of the first case suggest that the exercise of discretion on the part of the case manager is appropriate. She showed respect for the program rule by informing family members that the rule applies to them, apparently motivating their decision to have the older grandchild be the caregiver. When she discovered that the family had altered the plan, several months more had elapsed, presumably bringing the grandmother closer to the end of her expected survival span. Even if the case manager had then asked the family to revert to having Andrea be the caregiver, and if they had done so, the probability of the family's changing caregivers again was high. At that point, the case manager might report the family's nonadherence to the rule to her supervisor, and be advised to "let it go" or to arrange for another caregiver. The latter course would take more time, allowing the situation to progress even closer to the end of the grandmother's life span. Each shortening of her remaining life span strengthened the case for allowing the situation to continue. If death were imminent, the effort to change caregivers would probably be futile.

A rule that stipulates that a person who serves as primary caregiver of another be at least 18-years-old seems reasonable. Such a rule is based on the assumption that those 18 or older are generally more mature, and therefore more dependable and competent caregivers than those who are younger. But age criteria are notoriously inadequate in accounting for the developmental maturation of individuals. Moreover, even reasonable rules may be legitimately excepted. As Aquinas put it, exceptions are dispensations "of" (note, not "from") the law (*Summa Theologica* I-II, Q. 97, Art.4).

The case manager for Mrs. B. seems to have recognized an exception to the rule that was legitimate because it fulfilled the spirit rather than the letter of the law without impugning the status of the law itself. Seen in this light, her action was not bending the law but fulfilling it. Permitting an exception to the letter of the law was justified on this basis, but not on the basis of conformity to the traditional doctrine of civil disobedience. It may be that the rule excluding relatives under 18 years of age from payment is discriminatory because qualified young people are thereby rendered ineligible for fulltime work and equitable payment for that work. If the exclusion is *generally* discriminatory, then efforts to change it are morally obligatory; if it is only discriminatory in exceptional cases, then dispensations are needed to be applied in those instances.

The second case is less clear regarding the case manager's responsibility because some facts that would (or could) be known are not provided. First is the degree of need for regular injections; second is the possibility of a family member providing the injections; third is the relationship between the live-in, unrelated, paid caregiver and the client; and fourth is the meaning of "leaving it alone." Clarification on any of these points could lead to different resolutions of the conflict.

One way of showing respect for laws or rules is what I sometimes call an "ethical bypass" (Mahowald, 1993). It means looking for alternatives to accomplish the same moral end without breaking rules. Finding a family member who is willing and able to give the injections would be an ethical bypass that might introduce another positive element into the situation, namely, contact for the client with another person who cares. Determining the degree of need for injections is important because the risk to the client must be weighed against the risk of breaking the law. The latter is not solely the risk of liability for the case manager and her program, but also for others whom the law is intended to benefit or protect.

Determining the relationship between the unrelated caregiver and the client is relevant to the case manager's assessment of whether in fact the spirit of the law would be served by allowing the caregiver to give the injections. Presumably, an attitude of caring for the person is at least one of the reasons for distinguishing between relatives and nonrelatives (Noddings, 1984). Yet some unrelated, even unpaid, persons are more caring toward clients than family members. Discerning which family members do not or cannot properly care for their relatives is, in fact, an important obligation of case managers.

If additional information shows that the client needs regular injections to start as soon as possible, and that life or health would be seriously threatened without them, then the case manager is morally obligated to see that the client begins to receive the injections promptly by whatever means is available. If it is not possible to get a nurse, this would require choosing the person who would most expeditiously be prepared to give the injections, who might be a family member. If that is not possible, the unrelated caregiver should be prepared to do so—despite the fact that this is technically illegal. In other words, an exception to the law should be presumed, in accordance with its spirit. So long as the case manager is confident of the caregiver's ability to give the injections safely and effectively, as apparently she is, breaking the law is justified on the basis of obedience to a higher or more compelling law, namely, to save the life or preserve the health of the client.

The preceding paragraph had several important provisos. If these were to be stipulated differently, breaking the law would not be justified. For example, if the injections are a preventive measure rather than a life-saving measure, and their administration could be postponed without compromising the welfare of the client, then the postponement would be morally incumbent on the case manager to permit pursuit of legal alternatives. Only when such alternatives are exhausted is the breaking of rules morally justified.

Although rules may, and sometimes should, be broken in cases such as these, moral responsibility does not end there. For example, while the unrelated caregiver may initiate the injections, efforts should continue to find a legally qualified person to continue providing them. The fact that rules are broken because they are determined to be unjust does not eliminate the obligation to try to change them. In the traditional doctrine of civil disobedience, this is to be done by legal means such as negotiation, and only when such measures fail is civil disobedience legitimately practiced (King, 1964).

In a sense, the conflict regarding conformity to rules exemplifies the generic ethical dilemma faced by case managers because of their position as gatekeepers as well as client advocates. Rules, after all, are a means of gatekeeping. In either of the situations discussed, the ethical dilemma is raised by the fact that personnel who are qualified for the job are legally or economically unavailable. Moreover, the case manager is obligated to look at the impact of her possible rule breaking on other clients, and from a broader-than-case-manager perspective as well. Suppose, for example, the case manager is likely to lose her job if she breaks a rule, and suppose she is the sole support of her family and has little prospect of finding another job. From a broader-than-case-manager perspective, these are relevant moral considerations. In this complex world, professional moral responsibilities cannot practically be separated from other moral responsibilities that we have as persons who happen to be professionals. This is part of what is meant in saying that each case is different. Acknowledging our inevitable limitations in recognizing all of the elements involved in the complex ethical dilemmas faced by case managers can save us from arrogance and error in evaluating their decisions.

As individuals and citizens, professional persons have power that is intended to empower others (Mahowald, 1988). But responsibility in the exercise of power is proportionate to the degree of power in specific circumstances. Ordinarily, the individual professional has more power, and thus graver responsibility, to the individual client than to the larger community. The case manager is professionally responsible for a certain constituency as well as for individual patients, and as a citizen is also responsible for the larger community. This may lead at times, and appropriately, to a kind of "schizophrenic ethic." By that I mean that the case manager may make a decision to support a particular client, while realizing that the same support cannot be given—for reasons beyond the case manager's scope of control—to other clients who may be in greater need of such support. The case manager may then lobby to change the rules that would reduce her opportunity to care for the less needy patient for whom she currently cares to promote a situation in which the needier clients would benefit.

Breaking rules for moral reasons may be viewed as a kind of schizophrenic ethic because it suggests that there are two conflicting priorities pursued—respect for rules and commitment to the client's welfare. If the provisos outlined earlier are observed, however, this type of schizophrenia is ethically healthy.

REFERENCES

Aquinas, T. (1945). Treatise on law. In Pegis, A. C. (Ed.). *Basic writings of Saint Thomas Aquinas* (Vol. 1, pp. 742–748). New York: Random House.

Gandhi, M. T. (1961). *Non-violent resistance (Satyagraha)*. New York: Schocken Books.

Harris, P. (1989). *Civil disobedience*. Lanham, MD: University Press of America.

King, M. L., Jr. (1963). Letter from Birmingham jail, April 16, 1963. In P. Harris (Ed.), *Civil disobedience* (pp. 57–71). Lanham, MD: University Press of America.

Mahowald, M. B. (1988). The physician. In R. Lawry & R. Clarke (Eds.). *The power of the professional person* (pp. 119–131). New York: University Press of America.

Mahowald, M. B. (1993). *Women and children in health care: An unequal majority*. New York: Oxford University Press.

Malcolm X (1966). The black revolution, April 8, 1964. In G. Bretman, (Ed.), *Malcolm X speaks* (pp. 45–57). New York: Grove Press.

Noddings, N. (1984). *Caring*. Berkeley: University of California Press.

Plato. The apology. (1956). In W. H. D. Rouse, (Trans.). *Great dialogues of Plato* (pp. 423–446). New York: Mentor Books.

Thoreau, H. D. (1968). On the duty of civil disobedience. In *Walden and the essay on civil disobedience* (pp. 411–445). New York: Lancer Books.

Process of Legitimizing Rule Breaking[1]

■

Kathleen E. Powderly

These cases are good illustrations of the tensions that can arise between the case manager's dual roles as a client advocate and a system gatekeeper. Each of these cases is very difficult and leads to great stress for the case managers, the clients, and their families. However, they do not present rare or unique dilemmas. Similar conflicts arise in home care on a regular basis. It is necessary that the obligations of the case manager in such cases be prioritized to determine the appropriate course of action and attempt to resolve the potential conflicts between these roles.

There is a demonstrated need for rules and checks and balances in the system to protect the very vulnerable population served by home care agencies and facilitated by case managers. A long history of abuse and neglect of the elderly and disabled is evidence of this need. However, each case is different and, therefore, needs to be evaluated on its own merit. Otherwise the very rules and guidelines that are designed to protect the client may indeed penalize or harm the client. The two cases each present a dilemma related to individual circumstances that violates the strictest interpretation of the rules.

In the case of Mrs. B, a dying woman is being lovingly cared for by her preferred caretaker. There is no abuse or neglect except of the rules that prohibit the employment of a caretaker under the age of 18. Compared with situations in which home care is inadequate, impersonal, or even negligent or harmful, this is a relatively positive scenario. Would the client not suffer greater harm by being subjected to a strange caretaker in her last days? The family and the client are quite content with the situation, and there seems to be little potential for liability because everyone is in agreement with the plan. In addition, we all know that some 17-year-olds are far more mature and capable than some 40-year-olds! Mona, the case manager in this case, demonstrates the maturity necessary to fulfill her responsibilities. Thus, the choice of age 18 as the cutoff seems arbitrary. She probably gets more support from the family than a strange caretaker would. In addition, she receives the money that is being sent to Andrea. This case would present more ethical dilemmas if Andrea were keeping the money.

[1]The author acknowledges the thoughtful insight and assistance of Connie Zucherman, JD, in the preparation of this commentary.

In the case of Mrs. C, again, the client is being adequately cared for. Her basic housekeeping and personal needs are being met. She has simple medical needs (which are actually nursing needs!). It will be much more costly to provide skilled nursing care and would necessitate the removal of the housekeeping and personal care assistance to fit within the budget allocated. Thus, her medical needs might be addressed, but her basic human needs would not be. In whose best interest is this solution? The system would stay well within its rigid guidelines, which are probably designed, at least in part, to avoid turf battles. However, Mrs. C would be in real trouble. Every caregiver is not capable of learning the technical skills necessary to care for Mrs. C, and no paraprofessional should provide skilled nursing care.

It does seem that the skills necessary in this case could be learned by the caretaker and Mrs. C would receive more holistic care. Removing the resources that provide personal care and housekeeping can't possibly maximize health status for this client. If the goal for the client is to promote optimal health and provide holistic care, trading off one set of resources for another can't possibly help to achieve that goal. That tradeoff leads to promotion of the best interests of the system, that is, fiscal stability and reduction of legal liability. If one accepts that there is a finite amount of money available for Mrs. C's care, it maximizes the outcome for her if the seemingly competent caretaker is trained to provide the basic medical-nursing care. This is especially compelling because these skills would be taught to a family member in the same situation. This would help to keep the client in optimal health and as independent as possible. Denial of the personal care and housekeeping resources will probably lead to a greater expenditure of resources in the long run and can't help but contribute to a decline in health status. The removal of those resources could be the beginning of the slippery slope to institutionalization. This would be tragic and certainly not in keeping with the goals of case management.

Each of these cases illustrates the need for some discretion on the part of case managers. There is the potential for client abuse and neglect in each situation, although it is no more than a potential in either of these cases. It is in the client's best interest in each case to have someone responsible for playing watchdog to make sure there is no abuse or neglect. If there were no discretion, however, in each of these cases following the rules strictly would only penalize the client and cause more harm.

It seems that there is an obligation to see that the client's best interests are respected and that autonomy is respected. Changing the rules might lead to abuses, however. Each of the rules described in the cases was put in place to prevent serious potential problems. Removing the age restriction might allow a child, for instance, to claim to be caring for a relative. Additionally, there are skilled nursing functions and assessments that cannot be done by a paraprofessional. It would probably be better to make exceptions in situations like those described here than to relax the rules to allow situations that might lead to abuse or neglect. Thus, the obligation is to design a mechanism that would allow for discretion in exceptional cases.

But, what happens in the absence of such a mechanism? If one lives with the rules, clients might be harmed as indicated previously. However, not living within the rules does have some associated risks. In addition, if everyone *just* lives with the rules, there may be no impetus for change. There is the concept of civil disobedience and working toward change while living with the rules. This is a reasonable alternative to accepting the status quo. Each of the case managers in the situations described decided to bend the rules. However, when this happens quietly, behind the scenes, as it does in many situations there may be no change at all. There needs to be a way to protect the client's interests while at the same time highlighting the need for a mechanism to allow discretion in exceptional cases. Someone must play political activist to deal with the broader system issues. It may not be appropriate, however, for the individual case managers to play this role.

One of the driving forces behind rules and regulations for providers of health care and long-term care is the fear of legal liability. Liability considerations are important but should not be used as an excuse in situations that violate a client's autonomy or best interests. In each of the cases described, the client's best interests seem to be served by bending the rules. As argued previously, this should be accompanied by some efforts at a higher level to change the system and create a mechanism to legitimize discretion in exceptional cases—some sort of appeal process. This would greatly reduce the potential liability and protect the interests of clients. In the first case described there seems not to be much of a liability risk as everyone is in accord with the arrangement. If someone in the family objected or if Andrea were not giving the money to Mona, there might be more of a liability risk. In the second case, in which there are more stringent rules involved (i.e., licensing regulations for certain nursing functions), there is a real risk for the personal care worker. It may not be fair to ask a nonfamily member to assume this risk. There is probably more of a chance that someone will report this situation, and the worker and the case manager might both be liable.

In conclusion, there needs to be a way to legitimize bending rules in exceptional cases. This type of individualization is probably preferable to relaxing the rules, which may be necessary in many cases to protect the client's best interests. An open discussion of situations such as these, which happen frequently, should lead to a better balance of client goals and system goals.

VIEW FROM THE FIELD

Perspective From Indiana

■

Robert Hornyak

Rules are meant to be broken. This old adage may be better stated as rules are meant to be rewritten.

Many of the issues outlined in the various scenarios presented assume that all was going well until the case manager ran unknowingly into a new or inflexible or, at least, detrimental rule. Of course this does happen as new rules are put into effect, the condition of consumer changes, or new supervisors enforce old policies.

However, the daily business of case management is not at odds with these issues. These issues are important, even if 20% of the problems consume 80% of one's time.

Rules should specify the parameters of the ballpark, not define every inch of space within the arena. Case managers must have sufficient structure (i.e., rules) to

- Understand the applicable laws and regulations
- Appreciate the intent on which the laws and regulations are based
- Receive daily guidance in their duties
- Know there is substantial backing and support for their decisions

In any human service delivery system, no one set of rules can fully cover the thousands of possible interactions, conflicts, and exemptions that occur.

As a practical matter, 200 or 300 case managers, in a statewide program, cannot arbitrarily assign their own interpretation of what is in "the best interest of the client" and override written policy. Liability considerations are important. They cannot be so overbearing that they bring service provisions to a grinding halt. Yet, it is also accurate, without engendering paranoia, to advise case managers as to the potential risk of operating outside of established policy.

Case managers are receiving training on the rules. They receive less instruction on the actual process of decision making. Good decision making, use of supervisors, documentation, and the procedures available for changing or bending rules can be developed and imparted to a network of professionals. This can be accomplished before there is a "snap" in the rules.

EDITORS' QUESTIONS FOR FURTHER DISCUSSION

■

1. How much discretion should case managers have?
2. Is there an obligation to change rules that seem inimical to clients' interests?
3. Is there an obligation to live with these rules until they are changed?
4. In terms of the C. case, is the goal of case management maximizing health status, or something else?
5. To what extent should liability considerations guide the management of cases such as these?

Chapter 11

CASE MANAGERS AND PROVIDERS SHOULD BE FRIENDS:
Turf and Control in Case-Managed Services

CASE

■

The case management agency often has difficulties with its contracted home care providers. The agencies want to quit when the going gets rough, especially if, in the professional opinion of the supervisors, the client is unsafe with the amount of care that can be purchased. It usually isn't hard to get a doctor to agree with them and say the client needs nursing home care. Not only that, but if the client resists, the doctors are often too quick to say that the client is incompetent. They make those judgments after a half an hour of conversation, whereas the case managers often know the client much better.

The case manager has several cases that illustrate these problems. The usual problem is that the nursing agency tries to get clients in a nursing home too soon. But they also sometimes get too involved in giving advice. For example, she has a client with diabetes and open ulcers—one on the ankle of one leg and one on the foot of another leg. He was receiving personal care and housekeeping from one agency, and after the sores developed he was receiving nursing visits from another home health agency. The nurse had him hospitalized because of the ulcers, and they talked to him about amputation. The client wanted a second opinion, and the nurse tried to talk him out of that, saying that any doctor would give the same opinion. The case manager got the client an appointment in a nearby teaching hospital in an adjacent state, and the doctors there grafted an artery from another part of his body into his leg. He's got his circulation back and is doing fine. The nursing agency is really angry. They say that the case manager overstepped her expertise and went over their heads, and are not willing to provide nursing services to the client when he is discharged from the hospital.

Sometimes the case manager cannot decide whether the home care agencies are subverting the plan out of pure cussedness. She goes to some trouble to try to work out a schedule that meets her clients preferences for days of the week and time of the day. Then the home care agencies go ahead and do it however they please. They point out that they have an agency to run and that it is not the case manager's business to plan for the deployment of its staff. They can't get to everyone in the morning. The last time the case manager went head to head with an agency nurse on this kind of problem, the nurse said that she had discussed the changed schedule with the client and explained the need for it, and the client had agreed. When the case manager checked with the client, the client concurred that she wouldn't have wanted to cause trouble for anything as trivial as her preference to watch a particular television series. The case manager thought the nurse was overstepping it to appeal to the client, and the nurse thought the case manager was way out of line to plan the care in such detail anyway.

Other problems come about because the case manager is in close touch with the client and learns that the agency's worker is performing improperly, and is not supervised or corrected. Sometimes the case manager finds out that the care attendant is spending time watching television, or sitting and smoking, and that they are not doing all the work they should do. The case manager intervenes by explaining to the client that they need to be specific about tasks for the care attendant and that they should call the agency if they are not satisfied. The case manager calls the agency herself in situations that are glaring—for example, she knew of an attendant who kept "buying" things from the client and not paying her, and she knows of many attendants who bill the program for more hours than they really give. She understands that the agencies need to deal with the help that they have available and that these problems are not really their fault. It complicates things when the client also helps with the overbilling. The client is supposed to sign a log to say when the attendant was there. Clients will say that workers were there 3 hours when they were only there 1 ½ hours. The client knows it is wrong but wants to maintain relationships with the attendant. They want to be friends with their attendants, and sometimes they think the hourly wage isn't enough so they sympathize. If it happens, the case manager tells the client she knows about it and that it shouldn't happen again. If it happens again, she calls the agency. The case manager finds it somewhat of a dilemma. When she reports this overbilling and what the attendants are doing, she could ruin her relationship with the client. She also risks the client not telling her such things anymore.

As if it isn't enough to deal with nurses and nursing agencies, case managers also have to deal with physicians. Even though the program subscribes to a social model of care, the case manager has a lot of trouble contradicting a doctor. When a doctor says nursing home, everyone believes he's right. Half the time when you call up doctors and ask them to change a recommendation, they are furious. There is presently a situation in the agency that is even more serious. The case manager is sure that the patient is getting bad medical care. She's zonked out on drugs, and the case manager knows for a fact that her long-time family physician no longer has admitting privileges at the best hospitals. Her supervisor says she'd be crossing a line if she made a recommendation that the client get a new doctor. This is definitely not a social worker's prerogative in the supervisor's opinion.

COMMENTARIES

Strained Relationships: When Case Managers and Providers Conflict

■

Don C. Postema

The role of case manager is in many ways an *overlay* on existing patterns of practice and professional responsibilities.[1] There are both benefits and pitfalls as a result. The case manager can coordinate and monitor the performance of the various services required by a client, producing greater integration of services and assuring that quality standards are met. But conflicts between the case manager and other professionals are

[1]Rosalie Kane, quoting Carol Austin, the director of the State Unit on Aging in Ohio, notes that case management is popular because "it can be overlaid on an existing service structure, making it unnecessary, at least in the short run, to tamper very much with existing arrangements." Rosalie A. Kane, *Case Management: What Is It Anyway?* (Minneapolis: Long-Term Care Decisions Resource Center, 1990).

more likely because their roles overlap. Although the case manager does not typically provide direct care for the client, her expertise enables her to assess the quality of care provided by the direct caregivers; indeed, one dimension of her role requires her to monitor the quality of care. Her own relationship with the client and her role as client advocate may put her at odds with a caregiver whom she thinks is not respecting the client's values or wishes.

Ideally, collegiality would characterize the relations between the care providers and the case manager. Each would contribute his or her expertise to promote the best interests of the client, and each would recognize the limits of that expertise. Decisions regarding client care would be based on the expressed preferences of the client and would be facilitated by the consensus view of the caregivers and case manager as to how best to implement those preferences. Under less than ideal conditions in which the roles of the caregivers and case manager are ill defined or structured so as to overlap, collegiality remains illusive. If the resources available for client care and management are inadequate, and if the client's and family's preferences are ambiguous or unrealistic, the potential for conflict is increased. As the preferences and prerogatives of the case manager and caregivers diverge under these conditions, their working relationships can be reduced to a form of a "zero-sum" power game in which conflict replaces collegiality.

Seen from a different perspective, the case manager's role combines two functions that are typically separated in the American health care system, namely, patient advocate and resource allocator. The traditional roles of physician, nurse, or other clinician center on advocacy for the interests of the individual patient. The roles of the hospital administrator, insurance review officer, and program supervisor give high priority to the efficient allocation of available resources. The tension between the clinician and the cost-conscious administrator is internalized in the role of the case manager who is both advocate and gatekeeper; the interests of the individual client may conflict with society's interest in efficiency, and duties to the individual client may conflict with duties to other clients or to society.

Under ideal social conditions, the internalization of advocacy and allocation functions in the case manager's role would represent the decentralized expression of a society in which the needs of each individual were met consistent with a similar outcome for all others. In actuality, the case manager will identify the entitlements for which the client qualifies based on an assessment of the client's needs. The case manager advocates for the entitlements but may find that all of the client's needs are not met by the available resources. As the range of

entitlements narrows and the funding levels decrease, or as the resources available to the case manager do not enable him to provide
optimal care for all of his clients, the tension between his dual roles as
client advocate and resource allocator increases. The competing duties
to individual client well-being and to general welfare may seem irresolv-
able, and the role of case manager may appear to be untenable.

The conflicts identified in "Case Managers and Providers Should Be
Friends," arise under these less than ideal conditions. Collegiality
appears to be a distant ideal, and the resources to meet the needs of the
case managers' clients are less than adequate. Communication between
the case managers and professional caregivers appears to be indirect,
delayed, and confrontational, typical of relationships in which the power differentials are marked and control issues are close to the surface.
The first two cases are similar in that the case manager and the caregiver
differ in their interpretation of the client's wishes and best interests.
Ironically, it is the client who ultimately provides the reference point
from which the conflict is resolved.

In the first case, the hospitalized client is given one medical opinion
by the hospital staff (amputation for an ulcerated leg), an opinion the
client questions. His doubts are deflected by his nurse who, for whatever reason, assures him that there are no other viable alternatives to the
amputation. The case manager, perhaps because she knew of a medical
alternative to the amputation, perhaps because she was an advocate for
the client's right to a second opinion and adequate information to give
informed consent, facilitated transfer of the patient to another hospital
where an alternative procedure was performed. Both the nurse and the
case manager were obligated to act to secure the best interests of the
client, as he expressed his interests. Both roles, that of nurse and case
manager, emphasize the professional's duty to act as a patient advocate.
The patient considered it in his best interests to obtain a second opinion
and, by inference, to avoid an amputation. The case manager appears to
have identified correctly the patient's values and preferences, and to
have enabled their realization. Why then, did the nurse and case manager come into conflict when their role duties were nearly identical? Did
the nurse simply misinterpret the patient's wishes?

Given the intensity of the nurse and agency's response to the case
manager, it appears that they are angry not just as a defense for their
apparent misinterpretation of the patient's wishes. Their objection is
that the case manager "overstepped her expertise and went over their
heads," in short, their turf was invaded by an outsider who represented
a threat to their prerogatives. Had the patient advocate been a member
of the patient's family, the response might have been less intense. To

have an unrelated advocate counter their medical expertise and exercise physical control over a patient is an insult to their self-perceived integrity. Did the case manager do wrong?

No, and yes. In that the client's preferences were ultimately the basis for a successful resolution of his medical problem, the case manager's actions were justified. But given the exclusion of the nurse and the agency (and apparently of the rest of the hospital care team) from the decision-making process, the case manager acted unilaterally rather than collegially. If a case manager has a responsibility to those whose services she is coordinating, and if she shares a role duty with them to the client, she is obligated to enlist them in the decision-making process. A care conference including all of the providers and the client soon after admission would have been an appropriate forum in which to agree on decision-making procedures designed to respect the patient's wishes and facilitate their realization, if possible. A case manager should act on the presumption of shared authority with the other caregivers, recognizing their common duties and individual expertise, until that presumption is defeated by clear evidence that the other caregivers fail in their duties or in the exercise of their expertise.

The second case turns on similar issues and dynamics, but includes a reversal in which it is the nurse who correctly perceives the client's preferences in contrast to the case manager's interpretation. The client's desire to receive nursing services in the morning is clear to the case manager, though the grounds for her preference (not missing a favorite television series) and its significance to the client appear to be unknown to the case manager. Given agency constraints, the nurse-provider cannot readily accommodate the client's initial preferences and requests a scheduling change from the client, not from the case manager. At this point an additional client value becomes clear, namely, her desire not to inconvenience others for insignificant reasons. The nurse includes this value in the scheduling process and is able to match her services with the needs of all her clients. The case manager should be pleased, right? Her client's values have been respected and the necessary service scheduled. Where's the rub?

"The case manager thought the nurse was overstepping it to appeal to the client." But the nurse is obligated to respect the client's wishes as far as possible, as well as to allocate her services effectively. Appeal to the (competent) client to determine the client's preferences and to gain approval for a care plan is consistent with the nurse's role. The case manager's reaction appears to be based on the loss of control direct appeal to the client represents. Is her reaction justified? The nurse has a duty and a right to solicit the client's wishes and values. But the nurse, as one of perhaps several caregivers whom the case manager coordinates, has an obligation to the client and to the case manager to recognize that other services must be coordinated with hers. The case manager has the duty to integrate these services to secure the general well-being of the client, and unilateral scheduling by the nurse threatens this integration. The client has delegated the management of her care to the case manager; the nurse's duty to confer with and inform the case manager is an extension of her duty to the client. Therefore, the case manager's reaction was not justified for the reason she offered; the nurse was not violating limits on her access to the client. Her reaction would be justified for a different reason, though; the nurse's action, if it became a practice, would jeopardize the integration of the client's care. A turf issue, which arose in part because of the role conflicts between the case manager and the nurse, masks the moral dimensions of this case.

The tension between the case manager's role as a client advocate and his role as a monitor of the services provided is evident in the third set of cases. When caregivers or attendants engage in unethical activities which directly harm the client, the case manager must intervene to curtail or prevent such harm. (Intervention when an attendant essentially stole items from a client is a case in point.) When the questionable activities do not directly harm the client but are nonetheless unethical, it seems the case manager's responsibility to intervene is identical. However, when the client acquiesces in these questionable practices to maintain congenial relations with his caregiver (such as condoning overbilling by the attendant), the case manager's role is less clear. If, in addition, the suspect practice actually appears to compensate for a systemic injustice (overbilling to bring a substandard wage up to a reasonable level), the case manager may think any intervention unjustified. The case manager's role as client advocate appears to conflict with his role as agent of society, obligated to secure a fair and efficient distribution of available resources within the existing system.

When an unjust practice is deeply entrenched and unlikely to be remedied by any concerted action, compensatory actions that are themselves violations of the unjust practice may be justified. However, if there are avenues available to effect change in the unjust practice, such violations would be premature. In the current case, a systemic injustice cannot be permanently remedied by violation of that practice. Compensation levels for attendants and home health care aides are susceptible to political pressure; before these avenues for change are exhausted, individual acts that violate the practice itself are unjustified.

The case manager may be convinced of the foregoing argument in theory, but what's she to do in practice? Her client wants to maintain the good will of the attendants, which appears to be contingent on participation in the overbilling practice. Why should her client do otherwise?

Appeals based on the authority of the case manager ("I don't want to see this overbilling again or I'll have to call the agency and report the attendant") will likely impair her relationship with the client. The client will not let her see the overbilling again; he'll be more careful to hide the practice from the view of the case manager. Such surreptitious behavior may erode the trust essential to the relationship between the client and the case manager.

What's the case manager to do? The client may not recognize that he shares in the responsibility to use the resources available for his care and the care of the other clients of his case manager fairly. A discussion of the just community may be beyond the comprehension or interest of the client, but he may be able to recognize comparable duties to society he already accepts (lying to a Social Security administrator, taking more than he actually needs from a local food shelf, etc.). He may not realize that unfair distribution of those resources through the overbilling practice may put him at risk in the future for receipt of adequate care. In short, appeals to his sense of community and fairness, and to his longer range self-interest may be more effective means to enlist him as a monitor of the services he receives. If the case manager shares the authority and responsibility of monitoring with the client, if the client identifies his own interest with doing so, and if the client values the good will of his case manager, they may agree to curtail the overbilling practice. If they also press for changes in the compensation structure for attendants, they will be addressing the inequity at its source rather than attempting to compensate for it by questionable means.

The examples pertaining to the case manager's relation with the client's physician raise both patient advocacy and service monitoring issues. The case manager's role is an overlay on a preexisting health care structure in which the physician has traditionally assumed final responsibility for a patient, exercising the authority commensurate with this responsibility. The case manager's role parallels that of the physician in scope; she is responsible for integrating a range of services necessary to maintain the client's well-being. The case manager's authority is not commensurate with that of the physician, though; in the hierarchy of direct care providers the physician is unparalleled. However, both the physician and the case manager derive their authority from the client-patient. The competent client must consent to all services and therapies, and the client's best interests must be served by these arrangements. Hence, the client's autonomy and interests are a criterion by which the case manager's and physician's services should be evaluated.

When the case manager and physician disagree regarding a course of treatment or nursing home placement for the client, neither one trumps the other simply because of her role. Traditional physician role assumptions do make it difficult for the case manager to "contradict the doctor."[2] But the opinions of the case manager and physician both are to be weighed in the light of outcomes for the client. If the case manager opposes nursing home placement because her relationship with the client will end or be significantly reduced because of the placement, her judgments should be discounted. If she opposes placement because her client's well-being will not be enhanced by transfer to a nursing home, or will actually be diminished, her judgments bear significant moral weight. If the physician proposes placement because she has a habit of discharging all patients with a specific condition to a nursing home when individual patient differences may not warrant that level of care, the physician's judgment may be questioned. But if the physician's recommendation is based on a thorough assessment of the patient's needs and values, her judgment has considerable standing. The existence of a difference of opinion between the case manager and physician does not justify the inference that one or the other is immune to criticism based on an assessment of what is in the patient's best interests.

A different set of issues arise when the case manager questions the competency of the physician providing care for his client. Though akin to the case in which an attendant is double-billing in that the monitoring function of the case manager is foremost, this case concerns a judgment of professional competence with two significant differences. First, the case manager is dealing with a far more complex standard of professional practice in which he has far less expertise. Second, the physician's service is central to the client's well-being, whereas the case manager's service is more peripheral.

The grounds on which the case manager questions the quality of care provided by the physician to his client must be carefully examined. It is the client's relationship to the physician that must serve as the basis for the evaluation, *not* the case manager's. If the physician complies with current standards of medical practice, and the client values her relation-

[2]This difficulty has been experienced for years by nurses, social workers, family members, and even patients themselves. The case manager shouldn't feel alone in this situation! In defense of the traditional physician prerogative, it must be noted that the physician bears final responsibility and liability for the patient's well-being. Where other health care providers share this responsibility, less tension exists between them and the physician. Criticism is facile when one is shielded from liability for the outcomes of one's proposals.

ship with this particular physician and has confidence in him, the case manager has meager grounds on which to question the physician's expertise. If the physician provides less than optimal care but does not harm the client through negligence or malpractice, and the client prefers this physician, the reasons for questioning this physician's competence become more substantial. If another physician could increase the client's level of well-being but the client does not desire a change of physician to accomplish this, the case manager's duty of beneficence does not compel him to press for a change of providers. If the physician is negligent or malpractice can be substantiated, even if the client prefers the current physician, the case manager has a duty to end the harm being done to his client. The most stringent duty of beneficence is nonmaleficence; if the case manager can prevent or minimize the harm being done to his client, he must do so. The case manager's monitoring function then turns on the interest he has in the patient's well-being, and the dual roles of the case manager converge.

In these instances the case manager's judgments should be supplemented by other providers or family members, and generally should be confirmed by the client (the only exception being when the client prefers a physician whose incompetence has been documented). A care conference with the providers, client, and concerned family members would be the optimal setting in which to review the client's medical care. Review of current orders, medications, and therapies is appropriate, as well as discussion of likely eventualities in the client's future course of care. Decision-making procedures should be verified, and the client's values and wishes reaffirmed. In a collegial atmosphere where there is agreement on the ends to be pursued, discussion of the available means is more likely to be productive.

The resolution of the issues identified in these case studies turns in part on transforming an authoritarian structure into one in which reciprocity and mutual respect characterize the relations between the participants. Recognition of the expertise each brings to the care setting and of the limitations of that expertise engenders a sense of interdependence. The optimal management of multiple services for the good of the client and society rests in large measure on the existence of trust between the case manager and other providers. The integration of the case manager's role with the roles of other providers is a prerequisite for the development of trust. The case-manager role must change from being an *overlay* to being a *colleague*.

Charting of Clear Solutions
to Complex Problems

■

Joan Dobrof Penrod

This case presents several different but related problems that case managers face on a day-to-day basis. The case controversies center around interagency or interprofessional collaboration and conflict. The problems presented were complex, yet the solutions were clear to me. My views are guided by two beliefs: (a) legally competent adults have a right to make informed choices that society, in the form of professional and formal organizations, are troubled by, disapprove of, or see as the wrong choice; and (b) quality home care requires a healthy respect for clients preferences by all providers. Much of the case turns on these points. I will discuss each conflict and leave the one that troubled me most for last.

LESS THAN IDEAL PLANS

The first predicament described is a frequent problem for families of the elderly, case managers, hospital discharge planners, public health nurses, and direct service providers. The client is unsafe at home with the amount of services available to or accepted by the client. In the case, the home care provider advocates for nursing home placement and bolsters his or her viewpoint with support from a physician who judges the client to be incompetent after a brief interview. The client does not want to go to a nursing home. The conflict in this situation emerges from the different values and goals of the professionals involved with the client. The home care agency and the physician probably are worried about the physical well-being of the client and thus see nursing home placement as a way of protecting the client's health. However, the provider agency and the physician may concurrently be concerned about legal responsibility if the client falls and is injured or does not follow the medical regimen and overdoses on medication. The case manager, however, is putting client emotional well-being above physical safety. Thus, the case manager wants to respect the client's preference to remain at home even if an institution would be safer.

It is useful for all involved to recognize that legally competent adults have the right to make what some of us might consider bad decisions.

The preferences of legally competent clients take precedence over the desire of the home care provider or the doctor to protect the client and reduce their own liability. Just because a doctor says a client must go to a nursing home, the client does not have to go against his or her will. It is also true, however, that a physician can influence a reluctant client to agree to move to an institution but, if push comes to shove, as it may in these situations, doctors cannot force competent adults to move to an institution. Therefore, unless the doctor can convince a judge that the client is incompetent, the client stays at home with the best plan that can be purchased given the financial constraints and availability of providers.

Of course, this is all easier said than done. At this point, I would like to distinguish between the ideal solution(s) and those that can be implemented. I do not want to leave case managers with a "right" course and no guidance on how to make it happen. The ideal solution would be one in which everyone comes to agree through a group decision-making process. In reality, this is easier suggested than achieved.

In the situation described earlier (and again, this is for legally competent clients), I would try to bring all the parties together in a care conference with the client. Case managers will throw up their hands and say it is impossible to get most doctors to agree to a labor-and-time-intensive intervention like a care conference. Still, it is worth inviting the client's physician, and, if he or she does not attend sending him or her a report of the meeting. The meeting should achieve several goals. First, the client is allowed and encouraged to state their choice about locus of care. All professionals are allowed and encouraged to state their concerns about the client's decision. It is the role and responsibility of the case manager, with the backing of her supervisor, to indicate to all involved parties that this client is competent and free to reject the advice of the "consultants." A client who is informed of what the "experts" think is best and of the potential consequences of disregarding the advice and still opts to stay at home has that right. In addition, all the professionals involved need to carefully document the case conference and the client's viewpoint in his or her client records.

Finally, clients should not be abandoned by case-management agencies or providers when the "going gets rough." It may be necessary for the professionals involved with competent clients in unsafe home care arrangements to seek legal advice to clarify agency and professional responsibility. However, it is the role of both case-management agencies and home care providers, after an optimal care plan has been designed and recommended, to tolerate less than optimal home care arrangements to respect client preferences. This is a fundamental principle of providing quality care to elderly people in the least restrictive environment possible.

SECOND OPINIONS

The next case problem involves withdrawal of home nursing services for a client who, at the suggestion of the case manager, gets a second opinion before an amputation. The nursing agency believes the amputation is appropriate. This example is not an illustration of an ethical dilemma in practice, but it is a good example of bad practice by the nursing care provider.

Second opinions are a well accepted procedure in medicine. For example, in some states the Medicaid program requires a second opinion for surgery. Many private insurers want a second opinion for surgery. When a diagnosis of cancer is made, it is often the case that a second pathologist's opinion is sought. People are also routinely encouraged by health care providers, including oncologists, to seek a second opinion before cancer treatment. It should not be controversial for a case manager and a client to discuss a second opinion before a surgery. It is reasonable and appropriate: It is improper professional conduct for a physician or a nurse to take offense at a client who seeks a second opinion. It is well within the role boundaries of a case manager to indicate to a client that he or she is entitled to and might benefit from a second opinion about any aspect of the client's medical care.

Problems of the sort described earlier may be reduced with increased communication among the providers. The case manager, the client, the primary care physician, and the home care nurse should have discussed the amputation and the second-opinion option as a group. The client's interest in a second opinion about the need for an amputation would have emerged (or been appropriately elicited with prompting by the case manager) for all to hear. If the client wanted a second-opinion then the position of the true advocate is clear: help the client arrange the second opinion.

Again, I find myself arguing that case managers must be advocates for what the legally competent adult client wants, even if it makes other professionals angry. However, I am also urging case managers to take a proactive stance with these turf battles. Clients must be protected from interagency and interprofessional conflicts. Case managers should go an extra mile to preempt these battles by meeting with and talking to the direct service providers (ideally, with the client present or at least, with the client's permission) before the battle lines get drawn. Case managers have an obligation to treat all direct service providers with respect for their expertise and judgment. In my experience, this is a necessary and sometimes tiring part of case management. It means reaching out to professionals who may be threatened by you, or bothered by your involvement or who do not care enough to respond. However, in the best situations, ongoing communication with other providers, with the client also present and contributing, can reduce future conflicts. It is true that increased collaboration among professionals to arrange, deliver, and monitor care is time consuming. But so are all these turf battles.

A second opinion can also be used to deal with the situation in which the case manager feels a client's medical care is inadequate. The case notes indicate that a client is "zonked out on drugs," which is clearly a problem. We need not assume that the doctor knows the client is responding poorly to the drug regimen. The case manager (and home care nurse if there is one involved) might speak with the physician and explain the client's behavior, asking if the prescribed medications could be the problem. The doctor may cooperate and change the regimen. If the doctor does not respond, it is time to suggest to the client, or the family (if the client is too "zonked out") that a second opinion may offer the client a way to be medicated without being so confused or drowsy. If the long-time family physician is incorrectly medicating the client, a second opinion is likely to reveal it. In this situation, the case management agency should act as a responsible consultant, giving the best advice with the realization that the client and family may reject the advice for their own reasons. Again, clients who are legally competent have a right to make bad decisions, including choosing the security and familiarity of their long-time physician over possibly better care.

It is not at all surprising that case managers find it hard to talk to and negotiate with physicians. Physicians traditionally occupy a place of power and authority in acute and long-term care settings. They have come to expect deference from other professionals even when working in a social model of care. In fact, many physicians do not feel comfortable working with a model that does not recognize the preeminence of their medical skills. The case manager–physician relationship should not be different from other professional relationships the case manager enjoins on behalf of quality, coordinated client care. In reality, additional training and support from case management supervisors may be indicated to teach case managers to be assertive without being aggressive and threatening, as well as diplomatic, and strategic in their communications with physicians.

SCHEDULING

The third type of interagency battle illustrated in the case is over scheduling of home care services. A thorough assessment by the case manager should reveal when the client prefers to have his/her personal care and/or homemaker tasks done. It is also often the case that home care agencies report they can not schedule services to fit client preferences. Home care providers are not alone in setting up services to maximize efficiency of the agency at the expense of the client preferences. Families of residents in long-term care facilities and of patients in hospitals can be heard to complain that social workers are rarely there on weekends or evenings when they normally visit. I bring this up to dispel the notion that scheduling conflicts result from "pure cussedness" on the part of the home care worker.

The conflicts arising from the desire of service providers and their workers to schedule for their own convenience and efficiency is endemic to a variety of service sector organizations, including the phone company before the break-up of Ma Bell, the Department of Motor Vehicle Bureau when you have a question, and plumbers. Is the goal of efficiency less worthwhile than the goal of achieving client satisfaction?

It can be argued that there is a cost to the home care agencies and, as a result, to clients and society for the agency to operate inefficiently. In areas where clients are geographically dispersed, the cost of transportation to home care clients is not trivial. One hopes that the agencies *do* try to reduce those costs by scheduling visits efficiently. Clearly, fewer clients can be served with the same dollars if the routes are wasteful.

It is informative to consider that we have not empirically tested, in publicly funded home care programs, how important a particular schedule is to clients or how inefficient it is for agencies to satisfy client scheduling. An economist would suggest (and I agree) that a surcharge to be paid by the client for "out of sync" service delivery would help us test the importance of customer preference to both the providers who want the surcharge and to clients who have to pay for their choices.

Home care agencies should work for the client directly or through the case manager. In practice however, the influence the client or the case manager has on the agency is likely to depend on the degree of competition in the market for home care services in that area.

In rural areas there are few providers and thus, no competition. The agency has little or no market-based incentives to go out of their way to satisfy clients. In urban areas it has become more important to retain workers, of which there are not enough, than clients, of which there are too many. The case manager's role and responsibility is to find out what is best for the client, encourage the client to discuss it with the home care worker, and finally, to directly convey the preferred schedule to the agency.

I would argue that home care providers should be held to a higher standard of service delivery than is the person who delivers your refrigerator "sometime between noon and 5:30 P.M." However, I have tried to frame my solutions at a concrete level rather than at the level of demanding massive changes in the service delivery system. When it is possible to change providers to get a better schedule (and I realize it rarely is), case managers can help clients vote with their feet. Apart from this, it is macrolevel changes (e.g., introducing competition and innovations in service delivery) that will increase agency responsiveness to client scheduling preferences.

QUALITY ISSUES

Finally, the case outlines a conflict between the care attendant who does an inadequate job, the client who may or may not realize it, and the case manager who sees it all. When a care attendant "buys" things from the client and never pays, it is theft. The case manager has a responsibility to discuss it with the care attendant, the client, and the care attendant's supervisor to put an end to it. Rather than taking a unilateral action, I again encourage diplomatic and strategic conferences with all parties present to resolve this problem.

Do case managers have a legitimate role as quality control agents for home care services? Ideally, the client, the case manager and every direct service provider has a legitimate quality control role in the home care situation. In practice, it is often difficult for reasonable people to agree on what constitutes quality in home care. When the case manager identifies a deficiency, he or she should discuss it with the client before talking to the providers. Is it a problem for the client? If it is not a problem for the client and the care is also not negligent, abusive, or fraudulent, the case manager may have to change his or her standards. However, case managers have a responsibility to encourage clients to voice their approval and disapproval of services directly to the providers when possible and through the case manager when necessary.

The situation that seemed most murky to me was that of a client who logs in the home care worker at longer hours than the worker puts in order to "buy" friendship and loyalty, and also to increase the worker's hourly rate. I sympathize with the client, but there are consequences to the client if the fraud is uncovered and punished. Also, I am sympathetic to the underpaid, usually female and minority, worker. However, it is important to recognize that the services bought but not delivered come out of the services needed by another client. Rather than solving it, the fraud perpetuates and expands the problem. In this situation, the client's choice involves fraud, which is both illegal and results in waste of valuable resources. The case manager has a duty to point this out to the client and insist, gently but clearly, that the fraudulent billing must end.

In conclusion, the relationships among direct service providers, case managers, and clients are complicated and conflicted as are most human relationships. As a society, we deal with this reality by setting up hierarchies and roles so people know who is boss. What the boss says often goes. In this situation, there is often not agreement about who is boss. I believe that the client should be boss, and, whenever possible, client preferences should prevail. When there are disputes like those presented by this case, conflict-resolution techniques should be used. One effective tool is for the case manager to open or keep open the door for frank discussion. Additional training may be needed to achieve this goal and it may be worth it to case managers and clients.

VIEW FROM THE FIELD

Perspective From Massachusetts

■

Robert L. Mollica

GENERAL COMMENTS

The responsibilities of the case manager in these cases seem clear though by no means easy. Acting on them may be more or less difficult depending on the circumstances and the environment (i.e., are there multiple providers to work with or only one?).

The case examples describe a range of situations in which the case manager has to determine whether and what type of action to take. Considering first whether any action should be taken, the responsibility need not fall on the case manager alone. Generally speaking, the case management agency also has multiple obligations and responsibilities: to the case manager, to the funding source, to the program and to this client and other clients. The situations presented are real and not uncommon. The case manager should not dismiss them as isolated. If they are happening to one client, they may well be occurring elsewhere but have not yet been detected.

The options for handling the situations depend on the relationship between the case management agency (CMA) and the provider agency. If the CMA authorizes and reimburses for services, they probably have a vendor monitoring or quality assurance process that can be used. They might use the relationship between the case manager and the provider nurse, the CMA supervisor and provider supervisor or the directors of each agency to address general and specific problems. Relationships between case management agencies and providers should be constructed with a mechanism to review such issues that do not always force the case manager to handle them alone.

The examples highlight the importance of having good communication with provider agencies at the staff, management, and director levels as well as a process that deals with professional and client issues.

COMMENTS ON CASE EXAMPLES

Second Opinion

It seems clear that someone with less medical training has "threatened" the nurse by exposing poor clinical judgment. The CMA could use other provider agencies to serve this client, but the lingering effects may hinder the continuing relationship with that agency. The case manager could talk to the nurse and simply state that they had a disagreement but it should not interfere with the two agencies working to serve other clients. Obviously, this may not always work depending on the "egos" and personalities of the staff.

The case manager's supervisor could talk to the provider supervisor, acknowledge that it was a difficult case and explore processes to develop between the two agencies to handle future instances, should they occur. The provider agency may be receptive if they welcome or depend on referrals from the case-management agency.

Diplomacy is the key. The case-management agency might cite past instances in which staff has worked out difficult issues and areas in which case managers have relied on or welcomed feedback from the nurse. Agency staff need to feel they can express differing opinions based on their experience and judgement. Each agency has to value the expertise of the other if high-quality service is to be provided to clients.

In the end the outcome will depend on the history between the two agencies more than the conflict between one nurse and a case manager.

Service Schedule

The case-management agency has the role of assessing, authorizing, and developing a care plan that includes scheduling. Changing schedules unilaterally could interfere with the schedule of service from other providers.

Clearly, the nurse put the case manager in the middle. The nurse should have discussed the situation with the case manager not the client. The situation may need a management-level meeting to clarify agency roles or to develop a process for care planning consultation that may get the provider nurse's perspective before the plan is finalized without the case-management agency giving up their authority. The issue here may be rivalry, which may need higher level discussions.

Worker Quality

This situation threatens everyone—the case manager, the state agency, public confidence in the program, the provider agency, and its contract or license. Again if it's happening to one person, it's probably happening to others. At some point a client will complain and ignoring it increases the risks for all.

What can you say to the client? Let them know that you (the case manager) will handle the issue. Ask if they have any reservations about the case manager dealing with it. Explain that this has repercussions beyond each of them. Others may also be suffering and taken advantage of who cannot speak up. If the person is not receiving the full amount of authorized service, they are being short changed.

The provider agency's management staff will be very eager to know about abuse by employees. Generally, provider agencies learn about these issues before the case manager. They are concerned about their liability, their license perhaps, and their contract with the funding agency. The provider will normally deal responsibly with the issue and if they do not, further action is needed.

Process of Dealing With Physicians

This is perhaps the most difficult situation to deal with because the disparity in professional qualifications is greatest. The case manager could suggest to the client that he or she is aware they are having difficulty and knows the client has been seeing the physician for a long time, but believes it wouldn't hurt to get another opinion for her current condition. It would not mean the client would have to stop seeing the regular physician.

QUESTIONS

From a practical perspective as an agency administrator, subsequently I attempt to address the questions posed at the end of this chapter.

Responsibilities and Duties of Case Managers and Providers in Starting and Stopping Services and Relative Responsibilities in Arranging the Details of Care?

The case manager has the responsibility to initiate, modify or stop services based on information observed during visits, and information from family members, spouse, and providers. Generally, nonlicensed providers should report changes in a client's situation to their supervisor or to the case manager. Licensed nurses should initiate physician or other medical intervention as warranted by the client's medical condition and review the person's condition with the case manager. If the nurse's observation warrants a change in a service plan that is within the purview of the case manager, it should be implemented only after discussion with and approval of the case manager.

The case manager has the responsibility to manage the authorization. Providers are responsible for the quality of the actual tasks provided to the client. Effective communication is critical, but the case manager should have the final say in service changes and the tasks to be performed.

Conditions That Justify a Case Manager's Closing the Case and Withdrawing Purchased Services?

Case managers may stop services to a client for a variety of reasons, but they should continue to make appropriate referrals and interventions. The two most common examples where services are stopped are the client who cannot safely remain at home who refuses placement in a nursing home and the abusive, hard-to-serve client. Nurses and provider agencies may sometimes refuse to provide care when they fear their license might be jeopardized or malpractice charges filed if a client's condition requires more intensive care. However, the case manager has a responsibility to work with the client to identify and accept appropriate care. If a provider agency withdraws, the case manager should continue to work with clients who have placed themselves at risk. Case managers may not always succeed. Several specialized training and crises intervention programs have evolved to deal with such conflicts.

Honoring client decisions to remain in an at-risk situation is difficult. First, judgments about the client's ability to make decisions must be reached and referrals made to protective services programs when appropriate. If the client, otherwise sound, decides to remain at home, for example, rather than enter a nursing home, the agency's decision is more complicated. In practice, the decision to continue or stop services may be made by agency lawyers after reviewing their liability. This may be unfair to the client. Perhaps the CMA can develop a "contract" with the client when services are initiated that details how these situations will be handled. Such language could also be included in the client consent form. If the parties agree that services will be withdrawn when the agency determines it is not safe for the client to remain, at least everybody understood the ground rules.

It may also be appropriate not to establish hard and fast rules, and allow flexibility to respond to individual circumstances.

Responsibility of Case Managers Monitoring the Providers?

Case management agencies have a responsibility for monitoring providers, which may be implemented in a variety of ways including through the case manager. Provider monitoring falls into two categories: "clinical" and contractual. Case managers check with the client concerning the quality of care. They should talk with the provider agency's direct care staff or their supervisor about the client's situation to obtain their observations and from the direct care staff or their supervisor. Case managers should regularly monitor the appropriateness of the care plan. Provider agencies are responsible for monitoring the performance of their own staff. The case manager can note quality of care issues, but they should be dealt with by the provider agency's supervisory or management staff.

Case managers normally monitor the delivery of services according to the authorized schedule. Depending on the case management agency, other staff would normally reconcile billings against authorizations, review provider records and time slips, and check that appropriate licensing, required staff training and other requirements are met.

Juggling of Resource Limits and Client Preferences.

CMAs may be notified of a 5% to 10% reduction in funding, and they may or may not be given guidelines for implementing the cuts. In such instances, CMAs may tighten priorities for intake, close intake, reduce service plans, or combine these steps. The longer the agency delays in making decisions and implementing them, the greater the amount of the cuts that must be realized in the remaining months of the contract or fiscal year. These facts make it difficult to work with clients and their preferences.

Despite these constraints, client preferences should not be ignored and, to the extent possible, they should always be sought, discussed and honored. Clients, or their representatives, should be a partner in the care planning and monitoring process. As a partner, their preferences should be respected and followed. This principle often conflicts with the reality of service and funding limitations.

Criteria and guidelines that determine the allocation of resources should be established when funds are short. The guidelines may be established by the funding source, usually a state agency, or the case-management agency. Clients should have access to an appeals process when their applications are denied, services are reduced, or preferred services or the amount of services are not approved. Although shortage of funds is a real constraint, many states have not given clients due process in such situations. At least one state has structured the grounds for an appeal in a way that excludes actions due to lack of funds. Across-the-board or prioritized service plan reductions are examples.

In practice, the case manager has a limited role in brokering client preferences and limitations established by higher authorities. The case manager can always advocate for flexibility, alternative ways of meeting legitimate client needs, and changing of agency or state policy. However, guidelines can be developed that create a role for the client's preferences. If services have to be reduced, the client should have a say in what services are cut, assuming multiple services are being provided. Perhaps a weekly shopping trip accompanied by a companion or home-maker is more important than vacuuming every week. Or the client could determine which tasks take priority if homemaker hours are being reduced from 6 to 4 hours a week.

Even with tight funding and service reductions, guidelines can be constructed that allow the client to have a role in determining the impact on their service plan. The case manager may retain the "final say" and there may be reasons why certain preferences cannot be honored, but the case manager can ask and also explain the basis of decisions that do not honor the client's preferences.

Again, in practice, decisions must often be implemented quickly that affect many clients in a given agency, and require extensive phone and paper work by overworked case managers to change care plans, which leaves little time to spend with clients. Maintaining a client-centered system is difficult with shrinking case management staff, rising case-loads and budget deficits.

Physician Relationships to Case Managers.

The differences between physicians and case managers should not (though they usually do) create an unequal relationship. Physicians are at one end of the clinical continuum. Because of their clinical expertise, role and power, physicians often have influence over the type and location of services that are really the province of others. For example, physicians often prevail on placement in a nursing home over the case manager who believes (and may have better information to know) that an appropriate and safe community plan will work. Physicians often prefer a safe environment in an institution where the service is predictable and reliable compared to the community where services are less reliable and elders may be at greater risk in the physician's mind. The recommendations of case managers are often dismissed by physicians. Physicians' services are usually not among those authorized by a case manager, but physicians often feel their clinical judgments should control all the care and service plans provided by "lower tech" professionals.

While physicians are different from other providers with whom case managers work, these differences are more a matter of degree. The case manager still has a vital role to play with physicians. Progressive physicians rely on case managers, who actually see the person function in their home, for professional input on a comprehensive health and social support service plan. Case managers and physicians, when possible, should be part of a team.

Physicians can be too authoritarian in areas where they do not have as much expertise as the case manager, and they can also be too removed from the situation and ignore chronically ill clients who are served in community care systems. Case managers need skill and training in dealing with physicians.

EDITORS' QUESTIONS FOR FURTHER DISCUSSION

■

1. What are the responsibilities and duties of case managers and providers in starting and stopping services? What are their relative responsibilities in arranging the details of care?
2. Aside from death, what other conditions would justify a case manager's closing the case and withdrawing purchased services? Does the concept of abandonment apply?
3. To what extent are case managers responsible for monitoring the providers?
4. To what extent can agencies invoke resource limits to justify ignoring client preferences? Which type of client preferences are really important when money is short?
5. Are physicians different from other providers in their relationship to the case manager?

Chapter 12

PRIDE AND PREJUDICE—AND PREFERENCES

CASE

■

Case managers are expected to assess and consider their client's preferences in designing a care system. Sometimes this gets them into Catch-22 situations. For instance, they find out what kind of food the client likes, but short of cooking it themselves, they won't be able to get that menu on the meal program. Or they find out that clients prefers to take walks rather than to have their house cleaned, but feel they shouldn't give those priorities to the provider.

Sometimes the case managers really get into hot water on this business of preferences. For example, Mrs. J needs and is willing to accept care at home, but she is adamant that she does not want a black personal care assistant. She would rather go without care. The case manager, Mr. Jones, needs to decide whether to make an arrangement that specifies a white worker, or to tell the client that her agency is publicly funded and simply won't countenance such discrimination. He might be able to get the client to grudgingly accept a black worker, particularly if the problem is largely fear and ignorance, but if Mrs. J refuses then it is her problem that she doesn't get care. The case manager's policy is not to take racial, ethnic, or religious preferences into account when he makes a care plan. When pushed, he admits that he will make a special effort not to refer a client to a day care center that is under a particular sectarian auspice if he thinks the client would be uncomfortable with it. There's a day care center in a largely black housing project, there's a day care center in the Jewish Home for the Aged, and there is a day care center run by Catholic Charities, and the worker makes those referrals with a view to client preferences. However, the situation seems different from the one involving the black worker. Another client refused a Lifeline System because it came from a Catholic Hospital, and the case manager arranged a more expensive emergency alarm system from another source. Again that seems different.

Other workers disagree with Mr. Jones and would try to work around clients' requests for workers that match their preferences regarding race or religion. They point out that personal care is intimate and private, and compatibility with the worker is an important aspect of quality. Some would go a long way to help the client get a worker with whom they are comfortable. In the last resort, some would arrange a system whereby the program gives money to the client and lets the client find their own worker to circumvent this problem.

The issue cuts both ways. Many workers point out that they ask agencies not to send black workers to particular clients to protect the worker from unpleasantness. Especially when clients have Alzheimer's disease, they may lose their social inhibitions and subject the worker to racial slurs. Why not set up the plan to try to avoid such mutual distress whenever it is possible?

COMMENTARIES

When Is Being Equal Unfair?

■

Oliver J. Williams

The basic theme that underlies this case is, "Should you treat all clients the same?" In a society that struggles with the issue of difference, treating people "the same" or being "color blind" is often thought to be the behavior of choice. If one is comparing similar people with similar societal or racial and cultural life experiences, perhaps this may be a useful approach. When the comparisons are made between people whose experiences are vastly different, conversely, ignoring these differences has the affect of marginalizing the client who has the least status.

For example, European Americans have had a different societal experience in the United States than most people of color. Although history has documented the various struggles of immigrant groups, the fact is that most have been able to blend in America's so-called melting pot. Their ability to become the same has given them status, power, privilege, and access (Rothenberg, 1988). It has also shaped their experiences within this society. Groups that differ from the mainstream, however, such as people of color, have not achieved the same status. Historically, they have been forced to struggle, they don't "melt," and this fact has shaped their experiences (McIntosh, 1989; Pinderhughes, 1988; Rothenberg, 1988).

The present case highlights how status has shaped client experiences, behavior, and choices. Thus, the preference of a white client for a white personal care worker may have a completely different meaning than an African-American client's preference for one who is an African American. Yet when in doubt, some workers choose to be color blind, thus responding to client requests without considering the underlying rationale. It may be easier to deny the uniqueness of experience in this context than to understand it, but it is important to regard a client from the perspective of, "what do you need, and why do you need it?" The rationale that influences the choice clients make may be as important as the choice itself. Therefore case managers should not only obtain the "answer" from clients but also place it within a culturally appropriate context. For example, the case with which we have been presented raises an intriguing question but is one that has no general answer. As always, it must be answered in the context of the needs and personalities of the individuals involved. In thinking about it, it may be helpful to look at two possible variations:

1. The case presents the refusal of the client to accept an African-American care worker. But suppose the white client involved would accept only an African-American personal care worker, viewing the menial tasks involved as not appropriate for a white? Would this change how the case manager should respond? If so, why and how?

    One of the questions for this case deals with inequity toward the personal care worker. Does the policy adequately confront this issue? Would a client like the one described earlier be as likely to say or do something disrespectful to the personal care worker as the client who didn't want the African-American worker? It is clear that in both instances, the clients have a particular view of African Americans that influenced their choice? Both views may have their source in the same place, namely, perceived status differences and learned prejudice. Yet, are agencies and workers equally concerned about confronting these two perspectives?

2. In contrast, suppose the client involved were an African American who would accept only an African-American personal care worker in a situation analgous to the case as presented. Would this change anything? If so, why and how? The client may be concerned with how he or she will may be perceived, treated, understood, and accepted by a white personal care worker, compared with one who is African American. These clients' rationales are different, based on their status and shaped by their personal experiences of discrimination from mainstream people and institutions. Policies are set up to be "color blind" and "impartial," but this does not guarantee fairness. Nor does it consider differences in status or experiences. These two variations help us to see that our response to the case and to such incidents in real life needs to be contextual, rooted in a coherent value system and in an organizational structure that supports workers in reflecting that value system in their work.

ORGANIZATIONAL CONSIDERATIONS

From an organizational perspective, the following kinds of considerations seem to be important.

Agency's Capacity to Address Differences

The ability of a case manager to make good care planning decisions around diversity is influenced by the agency's capacity to address difference. Limited attention to this area will result in limited, unsophisticated, responses. Knowledge about recurring needs of a client population, increasing the level of ethnic proficiency, and contextualizing client problems will increase the agency's capacity to respond to difference. Cross, Bazron, Dennis, & Issacs (1989) and Leigh (1990) note that agencies vary on their capacity to respond to diversity, ranging from the culturally destructive to the culturally proficient agency. According to Leigh, in the cultural proficient agency, the culture of the agency and the cultures of population served are constantly studied and evaluated. These agencies conduct research on issues of multi-cultural service delivery and encourage staff to openly discuss experiences in multi-cultural encounters. Leigh argues that agency policies are but one factor in gaining cultural proficiency. Attitudes of staff, administrators, and clients need to undergo change. Practices need to become flexible and culturally impartial, and every level of the agency must participate in this process. An agency like this provides clear direction for the worker. Case managers do not rely on their own values or on agency policy alone; understanding and responding to client needs from a cultural perspective is encouraged. Organizations must build this capacity.

Staff Training in Understanding Behavior Contextually

Training is an important issue in care-planning decisions. Case managers must only contract with providers that have high training standards and whose personal care workers behave professionally. Among the topics that should be covered in such training are developmental issues including physical, mental, and behavior changes that take place among the aged owing to the aging process and accompanying disease. This information should help the personal care worker to contextualize the behaviors of this population. For instance, as clients lose some of their physical capacities, some may respond with frustration and even violence. Trainers should emphasis that, although the worker may be the recipient of such reactions, such behavior should not be taken personally.

Similarly, with a client who has Alzheimer's, or some other disease that lowers client inhibitions, workers should not take resulting behavior, which may include racial slurs, personally. Rather, they must recognize the influence of the physical malady and work with it accordingly. Finally, trust seems to be a fundamental theme in the issue at hand. Care providers must consider ways to earn the trust of clients, so that the agency service will be used as a resource by them.

An ethnically proficient agency will consider this an important issue of its responsibility, that is, building trust so as to be perceived as a resource by culturally resistant and marginalized clients (e.g., African American, Jewish, even majority whites, as portrayed in the case under consideration here). On the basis of trust in the agency and the case manager, the resistant client will be much more likely to accept referral to a care worker whom he or she might otherwise reject on prejudicial grounds. Case managers who have been trained as social workers are aware that one of their goals is that of advocate; accordingly, if agencies have not responded to issues related to client trust, case managers must insist they do.

DIRECT PRACTICE CONSIDERATIONS

In dealing with an individual client in the kind of situation described, the following are some of the kinds of variables that need to be considered.

Prejudice Versus Legitimate Preferences

In a "real-life" case like the one that has been presented to us, client preferences sometimes seem different from one another. On the one hand, people may refuse to have contact with diverse groups without any direct experience with that culture, religion, race, or sexual orientation. These persons may demonstrate anger, distrust, hatred, and hostility toward representatives of these groups. Although people and programs from culturally diverse organizations may provide needed services, these clients refuse them because of learned unfounded prejudice. An example would be an individual who would not accept an alarm system because it came from a Catholic Hospital. Such rationales are suspect, and workers should not consider them legitimate. The client may give them much weight, but it is important that the worker confront such attitudes, which are unfounded in experience.

Other clients may have a totally different rationale for their choices, even though the result, refusing services, appears to be the same. This rationale is the basis for respecting preferences. For example, there are clients who have personal experiences that influence their judgment about accepting service delivery or whose culture and tradition shape the choices that they make (Taylor & Chatters, 1989; White-Means & Thornton, 1990a, 1990b). In such cases the focus is on the effect of experiences or respect for customs.

In practice, of course, it may be hard to distinguish between acceptable preference and unacceptable prejudice they may indeed, overlap in a single individual. Again agencies and workers must understand the context of need to make the appropriate care planning decision. But what do workers know about various groups—the histories of the people and their customs and traditions? How do agencies facilitate that knowing? Care planning must reflect these factors—not only a mainstream perspective.

Many people of color who have long histories in the United States may, based on their life experiences, question the treatment they will receive by whites. Although they may be aware that not all whites are hostile toward them, history would reflect that many are. At a recent seminar held by Minnesota Area Geriatric Education Center for its fellows on minority issues and aging, a health care professional asked a Native American woman, who looked to be in her 80s, about the importance of having Native American health care providers. Among the things she noted in her response was the following:

> Based on the history of experience of Native Americans, trust is in short supply. It is important to have trained practitioners who are Native American or else clients would be resistent to utilize the service.

The right to practice their religion was taken away; families were broken up; language was disallowed; treaties were not honored.

This is from recent and distant past. Accordingly, these experiences will influence personal care decisions made by many other Native Americans. Another example of caution toward mainstream persons and institutions is experienced with many African Americans. Most African Americans in their 60s have directly experienced uneven or nonexistent social justice: Jim Crow laws in the South made it legal to treat African Americans with disrespect; and implicit or explicit rules promoted restrictions with employment, education, voting, heatlh care, and equal justice under the law (Rothenberg, 1988; Thomas & Sillen, 1976). They were restricted in where they could live, where they could eat, what hotels they could stay in, and the list goes on. In the North, treatment and restrictions were similar, although many whites fantasize that conditions were much different.

Presently, many aged African Americans note limited changes. They can generally eat and shop where they want to, but their life expectancy is shorter than that of whites and they are three times more likely than whites to be living in poverty (Center on Budget and Policy Priorities, 1988). In health, education, housing, and employment, however, things have not advanced much despite the rhetoric. Because of the suspicious and limited resources, many African Americans continue to use informal systems such as family, non-kin networks, and the church for social support (Gibson, 1989; Hill, 1989; Neighbors & Jackson, 1984; Taylor & Chatters, 1989).

Native American and African Americans are but two groups of color whose history and status shape their attitudes and behaviors. Dramatically, shrinking resources for social services in these communities are another factor (Liu, 1986, Liu & Yu, 1985; Sokolovsky, 1985). As a result, social service agencies must be inclusive of peoples of color; to do so, they must be cognizant of and respectful of the societal experiences of the group and of how history may influence preferences (Williams & Griffin, 1990). People who honor their cultural traditions find their identity and rules for living from these sources, which prompt decisions that are qualitatively different from those of persons whose intent is to devalue others. Agencies and case managers that have not developed the capacity to view the world from the perspective of persons with such cultural experiences and commitments tend to generalize from their experiences with majority clients (or their own lives), thus missing key determinants of client preferences.

Values Versus Empathy: Deciding When to Confront and When to Ignore

In the present case, one becomes aware of a struggle between values and empathy when asked to consider when to confront clients whose preferences are not "legitimate." The struggle is particularly difficult and poinant in the context of the age and the capacities of many elderly clients. At one extreme, focusing on values one becomes aware that persons regardless of age must be confronted regarding unfounded prejudice in attitude and behavior. Injustice must not be accepted whatever the age of the individual.

Further, to ignore the behavior of someone who, because of age, acts unjustly toward people of color or different cultural groups, would appear to be ageist and disrespectful. But helping professionals also depend on empathy in their work; from this perspective, one may struggle with the issue of confronting an aged person who is challenged by life and developmental changes. It often seems futile and punitive, although racism is wrong. But are we then devaluing him or her because of age and incapacity, if we do not confront this person? How sure can we be that a client's prejudice demonstrated through attitudes and behaviors are not life long pattern; in contrast, how sure can we be that such client's preferences are not legitimate or at least mixed?

From a different perspective, what is the worker's responsibility to "educate" clients? Where does this apply and where does it not? That is, when should the worker engage and challenge the client on issues of apparent prejudice and when not? A personal bias is to challenge injustice always if the person has the mental capacities to understand but this, too, often involves difficult judgments. Here as in all social services, trust building, is essential, as is discussed previously.

Confounding Factor of Available Resources

As mentioned earlier, an ethnically proficient agency would examine the needs of its total client population; this includes identifying what is common among all clients and what is unique to client groups based on race, culture, or gender. This clearly requires administrators, case managers, and personal care providers to understand the rationale or context of needs for these groups. Agencies that examine client needs in such a way are better able to make judgments around resource allocation and diversity. Further, such agencies do not assume that what is good for one client group is good for all client groups, thereby marginalizing the group with the least status. They are able to make decisions around resource allocation based on information and not personal judgments alone.

Unbalance in Supply of Workers by Race

What if all personal care workers available were African-American or if all were white? Under circumstances in which clients have few options regarding who the care provider will be, the process and resolution may be different than if there is a choice. This does not absolve agencies and case managers from the responsibility of being aware of the issues described earlier. Rather, administrators, case managers, and personal care providers, in such a situation, must rely on their knowledge of client groups as well as the skill of trust building to be more responsive to diverse clients with diverse needs. Further, this issue may have implications for personnel recruitment. Perhaps agencies should consider strategies which will encourage representativeness of both clients and employees.

CONCLUSION

There are no easy, blanket answers; each case must be assessed on its own merits. Perhaps workers are encouraged to ignore or to down-play diversity issues because they are expected to provide services to the largest number of clients based on available resources. If workers contract for services such as personal care providers, case managers may not have direct control over training, personnel, and the qualitative concerns of diverse clients about service delivery. As a result, agencies and case managers may question why they should be responsible for the needs of a few clients whose needs are different from the mainstream because of experiential and cultural difference. Why should case managers be concerned with that? Shouldn't the client accept what is offered or receive nothing? Benign neglect by case managers may be implicitly supported by agencies that expect workers to refer clients on a "color-blind" basis only and to ignore the diversity of needs. Ethnically proficient agencies and workers must study the best ways to respond to individual clients wants and needs; must be aware of the services that best respond to legitimate client wants and needs; and must insist on the development of culturally sensitive service delivery in contract agencies. To be inclusive, we must take responsibility as we respond.

REFERENCES

Cross, T. L., Bazron, B. J., Dennis, K. W., Issacs, M. R. (1989). *Towards a culturally competent system of care.* Washington, DC: Georgetown University Child Development Center.

Gibson, R. C. (1989). Minority aging research: Opportunity and challenge. *The Gerontologist, 28,* 559–560.

Hill, R. (1989). *Critical issues for black families by the year 2000: The state of Black America.* New York: National Urban League.

Leigh, J. (1990). *Issues in multicultural counseling.* Unpublished manuscript, University of Washington, Graduate School of Social Work, Seattle.

Liu, W. T. (1986). Health services for Asian elderly. *Research and Aging, 8,* 156–175.

Liu, W. T., & Yu, E. (1985). Asian/Pacific American elderly: Mortality differentials, health status, and use of health services. *Journal of Applied Gerontology, 4,* 35–64.

McIntosh, P. (1989). *White privilege and male privilege: A personal account of coming to see correspondences through work in women's studies* (Working Paper No. 189). Wellesley, MA: Wellesley College Center for Research on Women.

Neighbors, H. W., & Jacson, J. S. (1984). The use of informal and formal help: Four patterns of illness behavior in the black community. *American Journal of Community Psychology, 12,* 629–644.

Pinderhughes, E. B. (1988). Significance of culture and power in the human behavior curriculum. In C. Jacobs & D. D. Bowles (Eds.), *Ethnicity and race: Critical concepts in social work.* NASW PRESS.ISBN 0-87101-155-7.

Rothenberg, P. S. (1988). *Racism and sexism: An integrated study.* New York: St. Martin's.

Sokolovsky, J. (1985). Ethnicity, culture, and aging: Do differences really make a difference? *Journal of Applied Gerontology, 4*, 6–17.

Still far from the dream: Recent developments in black income, employment and Poverty. (1988). Washington DC: Center on Budget and Policy Priorities.

Taylor, R. J., & Chatters, L. M. (1989). Patterns of information support to elderly black adults: Family friends, and church members. *Social Work, 31*, 432–438.

Thomas, A., & Sillen, S. (1976). *Racism and psychiatry*. Secaucus, NJ: The Citadel Press.

White-Means, S. I., & Thornton, M. C. (1990a). Ethnic differences in the production of informal home health care. *The Gerontologist, 30*, 6.

White-Means, S. I., & Thornton, M. C. (1990b). Labor market choices and home health care provision among employed ethnic caregivers. *The Gerontologist, 30*, 6.

Williams, O. J., & Griffin, L. W. (1990). Elder abuse in the black family. In R. Hampton (Ed.), *Black family violence: Current research and theory*. Lexington, MA: Lexington Books.

VIEW FROM THE LAW

■

Reinhard Priester

As client advocates, case managers should ascertain and consider their clients' preferences in designing and implementing a care plan. By honoring client preferences, case managers respect their clients' autonomy. Client preferences that infringe on other people's rights, however, should be discouraged. When confronted with a client's refusal to accept a worker of a particular race, gender, religion, or national origin, case managers should try to convince the client to accept, however grudgingly, the repudiated worker. If the client's objection stems from fear or ignorance, for example, the case manager could simply talk to the client to try to overcome his or her objection. Listening and seeking to understand a client's fears and concerns helps build trust between the client and case manager. On the basis of trust in the case manager, a resistant client will be more likely to accept referrals to a worker whom he or she may otherwise reject (see Williams "When Is Being Equal Unfair?"). Or the case manager could try to persuade the client to accept the worker on a trial basis. But if the client persists, the case manager should overrule the client's request—except in certain narrow circumstances: (a) when honoring the preference is necessary for the worker's employer to perform its "primary function," and (b) when the preference is based on the client's privacy concerns.

CASE MANAGERS AS CLIENT ADVOCATES

An historical analysis of the concept of advocacy as a central value for health care providers may illuminate case managers' obligations to honor their clients' preferences. The traditional concept of advocacy required physicians, nurses, and other health care providers to advance zealously the interest of each patient or client, much as courtroom lawyers are recognized to have the duty to advocate for their clients. As one physician forcefully argued, "[health care providers] are required to do everything that they believe may benefit each patient without regard to costs or other societal considerations. In caring for an individual patient, the [provider] must act solely as the patient's advocate against the apparent interests of society as a whole, if necessary" (Levinsky, 1984, p. 1573).

Traditional advocacy also included the faithful discharge of care, the norm of doing good or acting benevolently toward the patient, a commitment to continue care once initiated (i.e., an obligation not to abandon one's patients), effacement of the health care provider's self-interest in favor of the patient's, and the view that the provider always ought to act in each patient's best interest—as the provider understood that interest. This view of advocacy, that the health provider should serve the patient's interests guided by beneficient paternalism, has informed the ethic of provider-patient relationships since Hippocratic times.

The changing environment of health care during the past two decades has forced a reconfiguration of the concept of advocacy. In the 1970s, patient autonomy, as exemplified in the establishment of the doctrine of informed consent and the creation of the Patient's Bill of Rights, began to replace beneficient paternalism as the standard for ascertaining the best interest of the patient. During this time the concern for patient autonomy grew to the point where legal efforts were made to protect the autonomy of persons who were especially vulnerable to impositions on their personal freedom. The health care provider's duty evolved toward one of providing the information deemed necessary by the "reasonable patient" to permit informed choices.

As the drive for increasing patient autonomy succeeded, the provider's obligations to their patients began to resemble what has become the contemporary concept of advocacy. Respect for patient autonomy replaced beneficence in society's view of moral priorities and the underpinning of the ethic of provider-patient relationships began to swing from trust in the provider's benevolent judgment toward respect for the patient's free choices. Respect for autonomy requires the provider to ascertain faithfully patient interests, desires, and values and to help patients achieve, whenever possible, what the patients themselves want.

Case management, regardless of how it is defined, includes client advocacy, which, in this context, refers to the duty to assure that individual clients get needed services. As their client's advocate, the case manager coordinates services from a variety of agencies and payment sources to meet each client's needs. In fulfilling this role, case managers are expected to assess and consider client preferences. Rosalie Kane suggests that honoring a client's preferences is the most important of the "ten commandments of case management" (Kane, 1990). At a minimum, honoring a client's preferences means spending the necessary time with the client to explain the array of options, giving the client the opportunity to review them and to select the option acceptable to him or her, and then respecting the client's decision.

BROADER CONCEPT OF ADVOCACY

Many commentators support expanding the contemporary concept of advocacy beyond the zealous pursuit of an individual patient's best interests, regardless of the interests of others. Critics of the narrow view of advocacy argue that providers have obligations not only to their patients but also to the organizations with which they are affiliated and to society. Therefore, they argue, providers should incorporate the interests of others when making treatment decisions for individual patients. On this broader concept of advocacy, instead of providers functioning as sole advocates of their patients' individual welfare, they would be required to balance a patient's wants and needs against the interests of others, including, for example, the interests of other enrollees of a managed care plan, of the managed care plan itself, of the organization for whom the provider works, or of society in general.

The health care provider's gatekeeper role in a managed care plan (e.g., health maintenance organization [HMO]) presents perhaps the clearest example of the broader advocacy role. Gatekeepers are expected to serve the patient's best interests, while simultaneously being cognizant of and complying with the plan's economic interests. They must balance the patient's needs with the managed care plan's institutional welfare. Although the potential conflict of interest is clear—to serve the patient, the provider may offer additional services; to serve the organization, the provider may err on the side of economy by restricting patient access to certain services—the gatekeeper function alters but need not undermine the advocacy function. The constraints within which providers must function (including, for example, policies to assure that a HMO's limited resources are fairly distributed among all of its enrollees) still allow the provider to zealously advocate for their individual patient's interests, albeit within the preestablished constraints.

While applying the narrow, traditional concept of advocacy to case managers would be problematic, the more contemporary concept is appropriate. Because of their peculiar role, case managers must take the interests of others into account in developing and implementing a care plan. Case managers can neither single-mindedly pursue each of their client's interests, nor honor their client's individual preferences, without considering the interests of others. Case management, as commonly construed, includes an administrative, or gatekeeping, function to allocate services according to their clients' (collective) needs. Thus, by the very nature of their role, in attending to the needs of any one client, case managers must consider the interests of their (and their agency's) other clients. In effect, the case manager must recognize that behind each client awaits another in need of services. Only in the imaginary realm of case management agencies with unlimited resources could a case manager zealously pursue each client's interests according to the traditional concept of advocacy.

A more controversial challenge to case managers' advocacy function comes from another aspect of their peculiar role. Case managers, as the coordinators, and sometimes the purchasers, of services also have obligations to the nurses, home health care aides, and other workers providing care to individual clients. An examination of the law may be instructive in analyzing these obligations.

Mary Mahowald (see chapter 10) has summarized the complex relationship between law and morality. She identifies five ways of viewing that relationship: (a) law and morality are the same; (b) they are distinct; (c) they may be at odds; (d) they are complementary; or (e) they overlap (see Mahowald, chapter 10). Another dimension is the relationship of law and morality over time. This dimension presents three options: (a) morality may change while changes in law lag behind (e.g., our contemporary views regarding sexual practices and sexual preferences no longer reflect our antiquated laws); (b) simultaneous changes in law and morality may be symbiotic (e.g., the recent emergence of the legal and ethical doctrines of informed consent were mutually reinforcing); or (c) changes in law may be instrumental in effecting changes in morality (for example, the 1954 U.S. Supreme Court decision in *Brown v. Board of Education* accelerated changes in our society's view of equal rights in education).

The last relationship is germane to this case. For at least the last three decades, court decisions and new laws prohibiting discrimination have been leading our country on the difficult path toward assuring equal opportunity. Thus, when a case manager is confronted with a client's preferences for a worker of a particular gender, race, religion, or national origin, it is appropriate to look to the law for guidance in examining the case manager's obligations to the workers who provide care. These obligations, most clearly reflected in the law of employment discrimination, restrict the case managers' ability to be their client's advocate, that is to honor their client's preferences.

EMPLOYMENT DISCRIMINATION LAW

Honoring a client's request for a worker of a particular race, gender, religion, or national origin is discriminatory under federal and state laws prohibiting employment discrimination. These statutes protect equality of employment opportunities and seek to provide equal access to the job market for both men and women and to people of all races, religion, and national origin. Under Title VII of the Civil Rights Act of 1964 (hereafter, Title VII), the most comprehensive federal anti-discrimination statute, employers cannot refuse to hire, cannot discharge, or "otherwise discriminate" because of an individual's race, gender, religion, or national origin, nor may an employer use these criteria in a way that tends to deprive them of employment opportunities.

Title VII's applicability is broad. State and local governments are defined as "employers" and thus subject to the same substantive and procedural demands under the law as private employers. Title VII applies even if the defined employer (in this case, the publicly subsidized case management program) discriminates in a way that affects the individual's employment by other persons (e.g., the home health care agency). For instance, a state department of elder affairs that was the defined employer was found guilty of discrimination in making referrals of home health aides to clients needing home care even though the aides were not employees of the department (*Baranek v. Kelley*, 1986). Given this broad interpretation, a case-management program would be regarded as the "employer" of the workers contracted to provide client service and case managers would therefore be required to adhere to Title VII's antidiscrimination requirements.

IS EMPLOYMENT DISCRIMINATION EVER PERMISSIBLE?

In some narrow circumstances, discrimination in employment practices may be permissible. According to the Civil Rights Act, assigning work to an individual based on her religion, gender, or national origin is permissible in those instances in which these characteristics support a "bona fide occupational qualification" reasonably necessary to the normal operation of a particular business.

The bona fide occupational qualification should be interpreted narrowly. Discrimination based on a bona fide occupational qualification requires a showing that a given qualification (e.g., the ability to lift heavy objects) is necessary to the "essence" of the business of the employer and that the employer has a reasonable basis for believing that all or substantially all members of the excluded group will be unable on the basis of the qualification to safely or efficiently perform the job involved. For example, an employer who wishes to define a single-sex job classification as falling within the exception must content that only one sex is capable of performing the duties of the job.

Restricting jobs to individuals of one gender, religion, or national origin, based on stereotyped assumptions, is rejected by Title VII. For example, many employers historically assumed, without proof, that women could not effectively perform certain jobs. Women were accordingly denied jobs because it was assumed that they have a high turnover rate; that they quit to mary or have children; or that they lacked aggressiveness or salesmanship; or because of fear that contact with customers or fellow employees would result in embarrassment or inefficiency. Such romantic stereotypes, general views as to the role of women in society and unsupported assumptions about the relative ability of the sexes have been rejected in our society.

The principle of nondiscrimination requires that individuals be considered on the basis of individual capacities and not on the basis of any characteristics generally attributed to the class or group. Stereotyped impressions of male and female roles, therefore, do not warrant a finding that sex is a bona fide occupational qualification and cannot be used to justify sexually discriminatory practices. Discrimination based on sex is valid only when the essence of the employer's operation would be undermined by not hiring members of one sex exclusively.

Unlike gender, religion, or national origin, race cannot be used under Title VII to establish a bona fide occupational qualification. Race is simply not listed as one of the possible exceptions to Title VII's sweeping prohibition of employment discrimination. This was not mere oversight: the legislative history of Title VII and the bona fide occupational qualification exception clearly evidence a congressional intent to exclude such exceptions based on race.

CLIENT PREFERENCES

The refusal to hire, or to assign to a particular job, an individual because of the preferences of clients, customers, or coworkers does not warrant the application of the bona fide occupational qualification exception. To permit customer preferences to determine whether discrimination is permissible would be to create an exception that would swallow the rule.

Nonetheless, client preferences as to an employee's gender, religion, or national origin—but not race—may be taken into account when it is necessary for the employer's ability to perform the primary function or service it offers. This exception, too, should be interpreted narrowly. For example, a hospital may acquiese to the demands of patients for intimate care by those of the same sex because failure to do so could impair the mental and physical health of the patient—the protection of which is the primary function of the hospital. In contrast, customer preferences for female flight attendants (allegedly because they are better able to provide assurance to anxious passengers, give courteous personalized services, and perform the other "nonmechanical aspects of the job") could not be considered to establish a bona fide occupational qualification because these aspects were only tangential to the primary function of an airline, that is, the transportation of passengers safely from one point to another.

A second exception to the general rule that client preferences do not warrant application of the bona fide occupational qualification exception is that client preferences for members of a particular gender, religion, or national origin should be honored if they are based on the client's right to privacy. In *Fesel v. Masonic Home of Delaware, Inc.* (1978) an action by a male nurse who had been denied employment as a nurse's aide at a residential retirement home on the grounds of his sex, the court ruled in favor of the defendant home. Most of the home's residents were female, who objected on the grounds of privacy to having their intimate personal needs attended to by a male. The court held that the privacy interests of the residents were a legitimate basis for establishing a bona fide occupational qualification. The court noted, however, that its ruling was supported by the home's inability to assign duties selectively in such a way that there would be a minimal clash between the privacy interests of the clients and the nondiscrimination principle of Title VII.

An additional reason for honoring client preferences based on privacy concerns for workers of a particular gender, religion, or national origin is that it may effect the quality of care, in terms of outcomes. For example, if the health care worker and client are the same gender, it might provide a basis for freer communication, including more self-disclosure. A recent review suggested that "both female-female and male-male [provider]-patient dyads would be expected to exhibit more favorable process and outcome attributes than would opposite sex dyads" (Weisman & Teitlebaum, 1991). Although the significance of this effect may be most pronounced in the uniquely intimate physician-patient relationship, it is reasonable to expect improvements in outcome (particularly greater client satisfaction) in other provider-client relationships as well. As the services become less personal (e.g., housecleaning, meals-on-wheels), the gender match between provider and client is less likely to impact outcome. In general, better worker-client relationships and better care outcomes would probably result if case managers honor client preferences to receive services of a highly personal or sensitive nature by a health care worker of a particular gender, religion, or national origin.

In sum, assignments based on protected group identity cannot be justified by customer or coworker preferences. The general rule is that mere customer preferences will not justify discrimination based on the individual's gender, religion, or national origin; however, a bona fide occupational qualification can be established by showing the preference is necessary for performing the employer's primary function or based on the customer's privacy interests. Beyond these narrow exceptions, a case manager confronted with a client's request for a worker of a particular gender, race, religion, or national origin should try to get the client to (grudgingly) accept the repudiated worker. If unsuccessful, the case manager should override the client's request, based on the case manager's responsibility to avoid employment discrimination of the workers providing client care.

REFERENCES

Baranek v Kelley, 630 F. Supp. 1107 (D.C. Mass. 1986).
Brown v. Board of Education, 347 U.S. 483, 74 S. Ct. 686, 98 L. ED. (1954).

Fesel v. Masonic Home of Delaware, Inc. 447 F. Supp. 1346 (D.C. Del. 1978).

Kane, R. A. (1990). What is case management anyway? In R. A. Kane, C. King, & K. Urv-Wong. *Case management: What is it anyway?* Minneapolis, MN: Long-Term Care Decisions Resource Center, University of Minnesota.

Levinsky, N. G. (1984). The doctor's master. *New England Journal of Medicine, 311*, 1573–1575.

Weisman, C. S., & Teitlebaum, M. A. (1991). Physician gender and the physician/patient relationship: Recent evidence and relevant questions. *Social Science and Medicine, 20*, 1119–1127.

Free to Be a Bigot[1]

■

Adrienne Asch

Once again, discussing ethical issues in case management brings together various strands of my professional life. Of all the situations presented for our reflection, this case causes me the greatest personal anguish.

For much of the last 20 years I have worked in various parts of the civil rights world, including 8 years as an enforcer of New York State's Human Rights Law. In that capacity I proposed legislation, wrote agency guidelines, and investigated hundreds of complaints of discrimination based on religion, race, national origin, sex, disability, age, and marital status. I am nearly as passionately interested in issues of civil rights as in those of bioethics.

PROBLEM IN CONTEXT

I am limiting myself to only one of the many points raised by the scenario with which we are presented. In the vignette, a case manager believes that it would be unlawful to honor clients' racial or religious preferences in matching them with people who will assist them in their homes. As I read this scenario, I had more empathy for the bigoted

[1]The author thanks Ellen Baker, Tamaara Danish, Jill Mazza, and Michael Rozycki for discussion and suggestions that have improved this article.

client than for the principled and beleaguered case manager. Although I might prefer the latter as a friend, I actually felt that in rigidly enforcing a policy intended to prevent discrimination, the case manager was engaging in another form of discrimination.

To understand my criticism, let me first enumerate the characteristics of the system in which the case manager, the clients, and the workers all operate—characteristics that permit prejudices to flourish. As I have said in my commentary in chapter 7, existing arrangements accord neither clients nor those who help them the dignity and respect they deserve. In this society, one mark of adulthood is self-sufficiency in matters of daily life. As soon as someone needs help to dress, cook, or keep clean, the person discovers that he or she no longer is regarded as ordinary. To others, the person is transformed from an alert adult into an incompetent small child who cannot manage anything at all in life. Often such people are taken over by health professionals, social service agencies, or unimpaired relatives.

The cultural ideal still appears to be that a person who needs help will be "cared for" by a husband or wife, son, daughter, or daughter-in-law who will have the desire and the time to help with shopping, cooking, dressing, or whatever else the person can no longer execute alone. No matter how resentful they may be about helping with these activities, family members may feel compelled to undertake them if only to avoid negative reactions of their relatives and the community at large. The person who needs the help often is distressed and ashamed about the loss of former capacities, and the shame is easily compounded by the process of seeking assistance from family members or from professionals.

Social services are available only after a government agency concludes that the individual's own circle is inadequate. A person must prove some physiological or cognitive incapacity, and then must reveal that she or he cannot come up with the methods of handling it. People who come to the attention of case-management agencies are less respected by the community than those who solve problems on their own. Much of the public regards the case-management client with mixed pity and contempt for needing help in the first place.

Unlike such government benefits as Social Security, and unlike a pension that results from previous employment, receipt of these services often is looked on by recipients and, sometimes even by the administering officials, as charity for which people should be grateful. Sometimes everyone connected with the case management process communicates to the client that she or he must toe a line, do what is expected, and make no trouble if services are to continue. In part this communication is unintended, because it springs from the recognition that there is not enough help available for all those who could benefit from it. Case managers want to feel that they and their employing agencies are doing the right things for the right people and do not want to put their effort into people who complain. The typical client, then, is often considered a marginal person who is expected to be relieved to get help, appreciative of the services given, and to have lost the entitlement to assert preferences.

The people who provide the day-to-day assistance to the clients are also considered marginal people. Because many of the tasks require physical rather than intellectual abilities, they are often considered demeaning and of little account. Much of the work can be done by people without a lot of formal education and is thus considered unskilled labor. Parts of the job, such as helping with toileting and bathing, can be messy, and the work is with "sick, old people," who do not confer prestige on their associates. For all of these reasons, in this country today the work done by a person who assists someone else with life-maintaining activities is not respected and is poorly paid.

The case manager who arranges the assistance, the person who requires it, and the person who renders it all know that the society finds it undignified to need help and unglamorous to give it. In this unhappy situation, with all its negative connotations, a white client refuses to have a black worker help her in her home.

PROFESSIONAL–CLIENT RELATIONSHIPS AND DISCRIMINATION LAW

Thanks to the laws designed to prohibit discrimination, most people now have some contact with others of various racial, ethnic, and religious groups. If we are mugged on the street, the police officer to whom we report the crime may be male or female, black, white, Hispanic, or Asian. A white racist may owe his life and home to a black fire fighter. We ride buses, trains, and planes driven by people whose race we do not know and might not like if we knew it. Our children's teachers or our hospital nurses and doctors could be of any background. These are only some examples of moments when we are compelled by the luck of the draw to entrust our health, safety, and welfare to people we might prefer to avoid based on religious, ethnic, or racial characteristics.

Most people reading these words applaud the legal and political changes that have enabled such situations to arise. We hope for competence and decency from people in positions of responsibility, and we believe that in promoting equal opportunity for all, employers will hire people who meet those expectations. We recognize that sometimes we will deal with people who differ from us in various ways.

Despite my support for equal opportunity laws and my desire for all agencies to adhere to them, I nonetheless claim that people have some rights to exercise idiosyncratic and discriminatory preferences in selecting individuals from whom they will obtain certain types of services. Let me try to articulate the situations in which I think it acceptable and appropriate for people to make choices that violate our notions of fairness. The question is: What makes these services different from all other services?

The answer lies not merely in the service sought but in the type of relationship necessary to enable the service to be provided and accepted. The client-professional relationship contains some inherent imbalances of expertise, need, and power. Laws and professional codes governing these relationships have been designed with these imbalances in mind and are intended to protect both participants, but particularly the one who is more vulnerable by virtue of seeking the professional service. To get the help people need from doctors, lawyers, or counselors, they must develop enough trust and comfort with those they consult to be willing to reveal personal facts and feelings. Of course, the professional to whom they reveal themselves must have the requisite training and expertise as well. Being comfortable with a tax lawyer may not lead to selecting her to handle a divorce or an adoption. But in seeking someone who can handle the divorce or adoption, people want lawyers they trust and with whom they feel comfortable. Because clients require another's expertise to solve a critical problem in their lives, they are in a vulnerable position and need to find practitioners with whom they can communicate and by whom they can be understood.

The laws prohibiting employment discrimination have been crafted to recognize the differing needs of clients and professionals in such relationships. Professionals such as lawyers, doctors, counselors, or accountants may not screen their clients based on race, sex, religion, or ethnicity. As providers of a service for which fees are charged, their offices and services are like other retail stores, beauty parlors, or lunch counters that cannot refuse patrons because of such characteristics. In this relationship of professional to client, the professional with the skill and service to sell is in the more advantaged position and may not lawfully refuse to provide help to people who have a valid claim to such assistance.

By contrast, persons seeking service may use any cluster of apparently rational or irrational criteria to select people with whom they work. Appointment availability, school of graduation, office location, sex, or race may all influence client selection. Generally clients who are dissatisfied with the first practitioner they meet will look for someone else with whom they believe they can develop a greater rapport. Their needs for comfort and trust are primary for the success of the relationship. As long as these services can be purchased on the open market, and as long as people can pay the fee, people are free to select a professional based on whatever they like.

RELATIONSHIPS AMONG CASE MANAGERS, CLIENTS, AND ASSISTANTS

At this point, I return to the case manager who is trying to find a suitable person to assist an elderly white woman in her home. On the surface, the previous discussion of professional-client relationships may seem irrelevant. The personal assistance is not being privately purchased by a fee-paying client but rather is being provided by a publicly funded social service agency. The activities required of the in-home assistant do not demand substantial education, specialized training, or particular expertise. Nonetheless, I would argue that effective in-home assistance requires the creation and maintenance of a relationship very much like the more traditional professional relationships thus far discussed, and for this reason, the client must have considerable discretion. Let me describe some of the tasks the assistant might perform and articulate what must go on between worker and client for those tasks to be executed properly.

Assume that the woman needs assistance with getting out of bed and getting dressed, cooking, and shopping. The worker may spend parts of nearly every day in this woman's company and may be the only other person in the client's home for several hours a day. The worker needs keys to have access to the home, must handle money in order to shop, must look in cupboards, drawers, and closets to locate things in the house, and must touch the client to help her transfer from bed to chair or wheelchair. Customarily, access to homes, money, and our bodies is limited to people with whom we have longstanding emotionally close relationships. Although the person needing physical and household assistance may be prepared to employ someone to do these things, she has no less desire than anyone else to feel safe with and trusting of the people who help her.

The frequency of contact between assistant and client, the privacy of the home setting, and the personal nature of the activities all suggest that the worker must not have characteristics that cause discomfort to the person she or he will help. Just this understanding of cultural notions of privacy has generated recognition of exceptions to the law against discrimination in work settings of fewer than four employees, and in housing if the owner would be living in a house to be shared with one other family. This same appreciation of privacy has also led to the recognition that a worker's sex may sometimes be a critical factor to successful job performance, as in not compelling female residents of nursing homes to be assisted by males or vice versa.

A satisfactory relationship requires more than the absence of characteristics that are disturbing to the client. For the assistant to be effective, she or he must differentiate the portions of the activities in which the client needs help from those she can perform on her own. The worker also must render the help according to the taste, rhythm, and mood of the client. The client must decide the order in which activities should be done, the clothes she wears, the food she eats, and so forth. The successful assistant must be able to understand the client's needs and personality, and must develop an empathic comprehension of the other person to ensure that the client remains in control of her home and her life.

Although the skills required of the assistant are not unique to a discipline or profession, they truly deserve the greatest appreciation and respect. Not everyone who is willing to be an assistant is suited for it, and people who will work well with some people will not have the personality and temperament to get along with others. The importance of client-assistant fit is recognized by many advocates for people with disabilities who support what is termed an "independent living" model of assistance (Crewe & Zola, 1983; Litvak, Zukas, & Heumann, 1987). They argue that client self-determination would be promoted best by having agencies provide the clients with money to pay for services and by having the clients decide who their assistants will be, whether they are relatives, friends, or people who answer ads to fill the job. Case managers who furnish the money while permitting clients to locate their own assistants need not be described as circumventing employment discrimination laws. Instead, they deserve a reputation for treating clients and assistants with dignity.

Even if the service system and all case managers were prepared to allocate money to clients directly and have them pick their in-home workers, not all clients would be prepared to undertake the task. So long as services primarily come through the existing structure, case managers and their agencies will be recruiting and training in-home workers and matching them with clients. This brings us to the client–case manager relationship, the appropriate process for matching clients with assistants, and the agency's relationship to the assistant.

Agencies assign case managers to clients expecting that the case manager, who is the professional, will work with anyone in the caseload. The case manager stands in much the same relationship to the client as do the doctors, lawyers, and counselors discussed earlier. The client needs to establish some of the same trust and comfort with the case manager as with other professionals in order to reveal her true needs to the agency. Although client and case manager may have only intermittent contact, the interaction must be more than superficial for effective assessment, planning, and follow-up. If the two cannot get along, the case manager knows that the agency should try to find someone else to work with that client. Applying the same logic to the client-assistant relationship, the case manager should recognize that even greater diligence and sensitivity are required in selecting appropriate assistants and should be aware that it is even more important for the client to trust the assistant than to trust the case manager.

Agency policy should routinely include a case manager's assessment of what characteristics the client prefers in an assistant. Case managers should focus on the needs the assistant is to fulfill, the amount of time to be spent, and perhaps some information about personal likes and dislikes that the client volunteers. Within the limits of the available pool of workers, the agency should take stated preferences into account before making any referral. Clients and workers should meet one another and work together a few times before a long-term assignment is made. The case manager should consider the feelings and needs of the assistant as well as the client in making the match and should not unnecessarily subject a worker to client abuse. As someone who gets work through a case management agency, the in-home assistant is entitled to be protected from discriminatory actions of the agency and its clients.

If the client believes she cannot be comfortable with a suggested person based on anything—personality or appearance, speaking style, ethnicity, or race—those wishes must be honored. It makes no sense to insist that a talkative client work with someone who wants little social interaction if a more communicative worker can be found. Similarly, it makes no sense to insist that black clients work with white assistants (or vice versa) if they have strong reservations about doing so and if other people are available. Case managers and agencies are understandably wary of honoring their clients' racial and ethnic preferences. Individuals have not been lynched or enslaved for being talkative as they have been for being black, and thus, the types of preferences are not absolutely identical. Our legacy of racism continues to deny people meaningful life. Yet, the particular client who needs help must not bear all the consequences of this history at the price of her own well-being.

Of course, the pool of in-home assistants may never be as diverse as one might wish in the ideal world. Until the job is more respected and better paid, many candidates will be members of low-status groups. The case manager may need to confront the client with the reality that remaining in her home may mean accepting someone who does not fit her personality or racial preferences. Faced with these less-than-ideal choices, a client may overcome her aversion to a worker of a different race and may discover that the racial difference is more than offset by other desirable characteristics.

Those of us who believe that positive contact between people of different races or ethnic groups may change even lifelong prejudice surely would welcome such a resolution. Respect for client preferences need not lead to complete surrender of such social goals. Initial assignments of worker and client reasonably could be made without awareness of a client's racial attitudes. After learning of these views and after discussing available alternatives with the client, the case manager is bound to honor them. The case manager may propose that, despite initial reluctance, a client try working with someone of a different race who otherwise fits the client's needs. If the interview and trial work period do not alleviate client apprehension, the client's decision must prevail. In the ideal world, positive contact would eliminate ignorance and prejudice. In the imperfect world in which case managers, clients, and in-home assistants find themselves, the difficulties may be too great. The client who needs help in her home should not be forced to be the victim of even a laudable social goal. In their own homes, even people who need help must be free to be bigots.

REFERENCES

Crewe, N. S., & Zola, I. K. (Eds.). (1983). *Independent living for physically disabled People: Developing, implementing, and evaluating self-help rehabilitation programs.* San Francisco, CA: Jossey-Bass.

Litvak, S. Zukas, H., & Heumann, J. E. (1987). *Attending to America: Personal assistance for independent living.* Berkeley, CA: World Institute on Disability.

EDITORS' QUESTIONS FOR FURTHER DISCUSSION

■

1. What are the limits on client preferences for their care plans? How far does one go to accommodate those preferences? Should cultural differences apply?

2. When does preference end and prejudice begin? Should case managers make those judgments?
3. What are case managers' duties and responsibilities toward the personal care workers and housekeepers whom they send to client's homes?
4. Should age or disability ever exempt a client from social policies or principles? Would it make a difference if the client were paying for the service?

Chapter 13

SQUEAKY WHEELS, LUCK OF THE DRAW, CLIENTS IN WAITING AND OTHER FAIRNESS ISSUES

CASE

■

As a case manager, Mr. Brown tries to be fair to all his clients. It perturbs him when a client gets a very full service plan when other clients who seem more disabled and needy end up with less service. This happens in part because some clients are so particular about things. Sometimes their health condition requires absolutely no dust, but sometimes they just expect a certain standard and have gotten used to it. Other people are so anxious to pull their weight and not take handouts that they struggle to get by with much less than they need. The program is supposed to try to spend as little on each client as possible so there will be more money to go around and Mr. Brown knows he shouldn't be persuading some people to take more, but the whole thing seems so unfair.

It isn't fair about family members either. If a family member is pitching in and giving a lot of care, then the program doesn't have to purchase as much. Sometimes Mr. Brown thinks this disadvantages poor people who tend to have large families in the neighborhood whereas more well-to-do clients have smaller families who more often live further away. Sometimes family members are just selfish and leave it all up to someone who volunteers. Mr Brown has a client who gets the maximum four hours from three days a week and goes to day care the other two days, but the only reason the client is able to stay home is that her niece gets her up every morning, puts her to bed every night, and is responsible for weekend care. The niece has a family of her own, and Mr. Brown wonders how much one should really expect of a niece. Maybe the program should try to do more (though they are pretty close to the cost of nursing home care already), or maybe the program should try to persuade the client to enter a nursing home for everyone's sake.

There's such a thing as fairness to agencies as well, and that has led to rules that say case managers should use a rotation system in referring clients to agencies. This bugs Mr. Brown because he has a pretty definite idea about what agencies will do a good job with particular clients. His supervisor explains that case managers are taking a lot on themselves if they decide to drive a home care provider or day care center out of business by withholding referrals and that the current policy is fair.

Then there's the whole question of eligibility. For clients to be eligible for services, they need to meet the income requirements. If you poke around enough and ask detailed enough questions, you will be sure to find something that disqualifies the client. For example, they may have too much in their savings for burial. Or they may have an insurance policy or small savings account that disqualifies them. Maybe they own a piece of property in addition to their house. As a case manager, Mr. Brown doesn't want to know about such things, and hopes the client won't mention them. It really bothers him that a straightforward, honest client who mentions everything won't be eligible for services, and someone else who has much less need will be eligible. Usually Mr. Brown will use his judgment. He had a case recently that stymied him, however. The client was a single man who owned a property that was not worth more than $10,000 or $15,000. He had nobody to leave it to, and planned to give it to his church after his death. He was adamant that he wouldn't sell the property and the case manager was frustrated because he did not qualify for the services at home he so desperately needed. Ironically, the church would just sell off the property anyway. The rules do not permit the client to just give the property to the church at this time either, even if he wanted to and then qualify for services. One is not allowed to divest assets to become eligible.

The programs also have waiting list policies that seem unfair. Mr. Brown has been a case manager in two states now, and he finds the whole idea of a waiting list to be a problem. The case management program promises to offer something to the elderly, but what good is it if the clients have to wait until someone dies or drops out of the program even to get their assessment? He is sure that there are people on the caseloads whose needs are less than those on the waiting lists, though it is hard to tell that when a formal assessment is not done. In the state where he previously worked, each county case-management program was expected to serve a certain percentage of older clients and younger handicapped clients. In his view, this led to unconscionable failure to serve the elderly in a timely way.

COMMENTARIES

Fairness and the Squeaking Wheel
of (Mis)Fortune

■

Steven H. Miles

There is no justice in sickness or human need. There is little justice in the way that family resources of cash, caregivers, location match up with the services of human services agencies. Some families have ideal caregivers, people of limitless energy, kindness, and skill. Other persons are without families or have families who are unable or unwilling to even do the minor tasks that make the crucial difference.

There is also little justice in our feelings to clients. There are clients and families that human service workers just "click" with; there are clients who are disliked, hated, and avoided. We incorporate these feelings in our conclusions about who is "getting enough," who is being "let off the hook," who is "not doing their share," and who "needs" the extra effort to rescue them. These interpersonal realities pose an issue for fairness. There is no easy way to resolve the interplay of feelings and circumstances in the fair provision of human services. Exceptions based on "exceptional circumstances" can be arbitrary, administratively unworkable, and overly influenced by personal feelings and judgments which ought to be irrelevant. Going "by the book" can be unfair to those with special situations. Every rule needs an exception; every loophole begs for a rule.

The fit between human service programs and individual needs is an uncomfortable one. Policies, however flexible, are designed for the purely hypothetical "average" client. Institutional services are never as intimately knowledgeable or individually tailored as the personal problems they would address. Human services can never fairly adjust for the uneven distribution of resources and problems of clients and families. There are not enough ways to help some clients. Other clients, with lesser needs and greater personal, familial or interpersonal resources, are adequately, sometimes even lavishly, served.

And to top it all off, somewhere in virtually every human service office there is a well intentioned but infuriatingly misworded plaque on a worker's desk,

> Grant me the serenity to accept the things I can not change,
> the courage to change those I can,
> and the wisdom to know the difference.

Serenity is a bureaucrat's most infuriating indulgence: "I'm sorry, those are the rules."

Fairness is a complex challenge for case managers. In its simplest form, fairness means that people with comparable needs should be equally serviced. A somewhat contradictory definition says that human services must compensate for life's misfortunes by providing more aid, more readily to those who are more burdened so as to compensate for the disadvantages they endure. There is no single or easy idea of fairness for the highly individualized and complex task of case management which tells how to have equitable general policies with fair exceptions.

Fairness can be advanced by three rules which I illustrate with several types of specific case management problems.

Rule 1. When a Social Service Meets Emergency Needs, Those Needs in which the Patient's Welfare is Imminently Endangered, Considerable Flexibility to General Rules must be Allowed.

This rule is examined by considering enrollment policies. Fair enrollment policies depend on the nature of the service and whether the service's mission is to meet a community need or serve individuals.

1. Programs that offer services in response to a client's own identification of need can be served by a first-come, first-served waiting list. For example, access to taxis for mobility impaired persons can be handled by a phone line with open reservations.
2. Outreach programs that are responsible for identifying clients with emergency needs should develop referral networks, enrollment priorities, and screening procedures to proactively engage

community groups most likely to need the service. For example, programs to prevent child abuse or neglect might be aimed to especially contact parents who are previous abusers, psychiatrically ill, chemically dependent, young, indigent, or unmarried depending on the known patterns of child abuse in that community.

3. Programs that address persons with emergency needs and those with less critical needs, may fairly terminate or limit services as necessary in order to meet the emergency needs of other underserved persons. For example, during cold winters, procedures for providing housing should focus on persons at risk of being in unheated dwellings over the needs of relocating disabled persons to handicap-accessible buildings.

All of these examples for fair enrollment rest on a clear definition of the mission of the human service program. Programs that exist simply to provide individually requested services rather than to address a problem for the community will tend to favor squeaky wheels. Outreach programs must ensure that enrollment procedures are "skewed" to favor wheels that are falling off rather than those who are simply squeaky. Eligible, currently serviced clients may even be terminated by fair procedures when other eligible persons have emergency needs.

Many human service programs have missions to serve clients with emergency and non-emergency needs. For example, an adult day care program might meet the needs of caregivers in crisis as well as those who want a place for a demented mother to spend the day so that the caregiver can lead a life outside the home. Enrollment policies might reserve 5 of forty openings for emergency enrollments. If over time it appears that ten slots are needed for emergency respite; the frequency of service to less needy clients may be cut. The admission contract to non-emergency enrollees should describe this possibility.

Rule 2. Fairness to Clients' Needs Preempts Fairness to Providers.

There is no duty to share referrals of clients with multiple providers fairly. Thus, there is no need to rotate referrals among several providers so they might profit equally. Rotation might well be done for reasons that served clients' interests. The only obligations pertain to avoiding fee splitting as a cartel, or maliciously acting to destroy a provider's business. Providers should be selected because they best serve the client's needs. Consider the following application of the rule:

A hospital refers patients to five nursing homes. Facility 1 is known by social workers to have problems with quality control. Facility 2 is 10 miles outside of town. A smaller facility 3 has only one nurse who can perform admission workups. The last three nursing home placements have gone to facilities 4 and 5. Two hospital inpatients are being discharged to nursing homes on a Friday before a 3-day weekend. If sending both patients to facility 3 would result in an inadequate workup before the weekend, then it would be appropriate to send no more than one patient to facility 3. The family of a nursing home resident should not be burdened with an extra 10 miles of distance to a facility 2 simply to ensure an equal use of facilities. It would be inappropriate to boycott facility 1, but there is no obligation to use facility 1 simply because of a need to equally rotate patients, though it may be appropriate to send patients there for other reasons. Facilities 4 and 5 should not be disqualified because they have been most recently used.

Rule 3. Fairness Sometime Requires a Human Interpretation of the Intent, rather than the Letter, of Human Service Policies.

Policies can be "tweaked" when their rigidity seems to be unfair in application to an unusual client whom the program is supposed to serve. Consider the following scenario:

A county adult day care program is designed to meet the needs of caregivers of disabled elderly. It offers a full day program at full price and a 4-hour morning or afternoon programs at half price. A woman who lives with her demented father works the business lunch shift as a short order cook. He becomes unsafe to leave at home. She cannot afford the sliding scale full day rate but would like to leave him for 4 hours in the middle of the day. The case manager gets the center to agree to a half day rate.

Exemptions should not be granted for regulations whose injustice falls evenly on all. Regulations should be administered according to their intent. These call for political reform, not maverick case work. Again an example.

Medicare does not cover screening mammograms for anyone but does cover mammograms that are used to investigate suspicious lumps in the breast. An indigent 66 year old woman has not had a mammogram. The public nurse should not ask the doctor to write "evaluate mass" on the mammogram request for one of her favorite clients so that she can get a free mammogram.

Fairness has a contradiction in it. Case managers need uniform policies to treat comparable needs comparably. They also need an eye for the legitimate exception to fairly respond to exceptional circumstances. Fairness involves tradeoffs between the conflicting responsibility to play by the book and to advocate for our clients. Case management requires fortitude to work within constraints on behalf of needy clients. Case managers should measure the quality of their work by how well they have been advocates for their clients and how well they have supported fundamental policy reform to meet clients' needs, rather than by how well they have met the procedural requirements of their job. Case managers could use a new plaque.

> Grant me the courage to bear the things I can not change,
> the serenity to change those I can,
> and the smarts to know what's what.

Can Familial Caregiving Be Required?

■

Stephen G. Post

Mr. Brown is a case manager concerned with fairness or justice. When resources are seriously limited, and when people in genuine need of care management have insufficient access as a result, the care manager must inevitably attempt to distribute services as fairly as possible. I will focus on Mr. Brown's concerns with clients whose families refuse to care directly and therefore cost the case-management program more than is the case with clients whose families do caregiving.

FAMILY CAREGIVING

Family caregiving is a complicated matter. Daughters and daughters-in-law are typically called on to provide emotional support and assistance for those needing long-term care. Over the last decade, national attention has focused on "women in the middle," on women sandwiched between job and family duties. The extension of the human life span means that "contemporary adult children provide more care and more difficult care to more parents and parents-in-law over much longer periods of time than has ever been the case before." Studies indicate that women outnumber men as the care givers for disabled parents by a ratio of 4 to 1 (Brody, 1990, p. 35). Although results vary somewhat, studies also indicate that about half these women experience stress in the form of depression, sleeplessness, anger, and emotional exhaustion.

Historian Ann Douglas has examined the ideal of "disinterested benevolence" in American cultural history. She voices suspicion of an ideal that seems to assume that women have no needs of their own but serve others "for the world's comfort" (Douglas, 1977, p. 50). Such images of women leave them outside the domain of justice, for radical self-denial allows the agent no interests to assert over against the needs of others. Even contemporary feminist ethicists who affirm the importance of caregiving are quick to point out that "care" should not be defined in terms of radical self-denial, and that the caregiver is in need of care herself.

The danger of an ethic of care is a too extreme restraint on self-assertion in the effort to achieve complete disinterestedness. Any policy that requires such restraint easily becomes morbid, and may make for injustice by encouraging undue self-assertion in others. It is imperative for care managers to think through an adequate definition of the caring ethic, one that accounts for the direct or "first-order" desires of the caregiver with respect to career interests, entertainment, and so on, and one that supports "second-order" desires or inclinations to care for the needs of others with respite. I borrow this distinction between first- and second-order desires from Rawls (1971).

Case managers should understand the realities of family caregiver burnout, and should intervene to prevent this. Family care giving is a precious moral resource, and therefore deserves protection. The surest way to weaken this resource is to overwhelm it. This note of caution should not be interpreted as antifamilial. With the communitarians, I want to encourage reciprocal caring within the familial domain, but with some reasonable sense of limits.

Precise limits on family care giving will depend on individual circumstances. Emotional, cultural, religious, and other factors will determine the extent and limits of care giving. A case manager must pay attention to the particular case at hand. There is no need to argue about the precise point at which the burden of caring becomes unsustainable for the niece who concerns Mr. Brown. Rather, the proportions of the problem should be recognized, and programs to mitigate it emphasized. If family members wish to provide care that is often uniquely beneficial, then it is poor case management to press them to the point of exhaustion where in desperation, they surrender a parent, spouse, or child to an institution. Then everyone loses.

Mr. Brown is right to be concerned about the niece, who has a family of her own. She puts the client to bed each night, gets her up each morning, and is responsible for weekend care. The key element, though, is how the niece interprets this commitment morally, and perhaps religiously. Caregivers are an extremely heterogeneous group, allowing no clear policies to be developed. Regarding large extended families that are willing to delegate care giving tasks, this is pure gain.

It is necessary to avoid labeling family members who refuse to care as selfish. In one case I am familiar with, a 62-year-old woman brought her demented 84-year-old father into the elder health care center for a dementia assessment. She revealed to the physician that as a young girl, her father had raped her repeatedly. As a daughter, she proclaimed, she owed him absolutely nothing and refused to provide care. She only brought him in because her siblings were in other parts of the country, and she would not bring him in again. She only did so this one time, and only because her father is a human being. In other words, she assisted him not as a daughter would assist a father who had cared reasonably well for his children but rather as one stranger to another. She insisted that she would have done the same had she encountered some demented and lost old man on the street corner.

It was, in my view, remarkable that this woman attended to her father at all. She certainly had no filial duties to him, because he had failed so miserably to fulfill parental obligations consistent with the general standards of our culture. To force this woman to be a caregiver would result in substandard care, abuse of the client, and even deeper resentment.

The case manager must deal with disparity when it comes to encouraging familial caring. Sometimes, while family caregiving will save money for the management program, it is unethical because it imposes on someone who for good reason either refuses to care, or who cannot care without sacrificing self to inordinate degrees (Post, 1990). It is best to let each case situation resolve itself according to its unique features. In this moral domain, there are no equalitarian solutions. Fairness is highly illusive. There would certainly be instances in which a case manager is obligated to rescue a family caregiver even though the costs to the program might increase. In some cases, family care giving might be encouraged and training programs for family caregivers offered.

BASIC CARE PLAN

Mr. Brown is concerned with clients who, because of life-style, desire a service plan of a higher standard than seems objectively called for. He is also concerned with clients who are anxious to pull their own weight, and therefore struggle to get by with less than they need. This raises the question of whether similar levels of disability require similar care plans. Excessive use of limited resources is unfair, and ought to be discouraged. Basic care packages specific to degrees of disability could be developed and implemented, although dissatisfaction from those whose life-style is costly is inevitable.

Those clients who try to get by with less than a basic package may do so, since we cannot force those who competently refuse goods to accept them. A case manager, however, should try to convince such clients that there is nothing shameful or wrong with being dependent on the help of others. Both groups of clients struggle with individualism: those who overuse resources need to be informed that goods are limited; those who underuse resources need to know that receiving needed support is just.

Those who refuse necessary services may interpret dependence on others as unreasonable or burdensome imposition. They need to be reminded that human beings are dependent on one another. In a culture that emphasizes autonomy, rights, and independence, it is essential to recognize our inherent dependence on others, and the reality of human fragility. How hard should a case manager press a client to accept more extensive services? It is reasonable to attempt persuasion, but ultimately, respect for the self-determination of the recipients of care is essential. It is easy to overlook the importance of choice in the context of routine, everyday matters. Clients may well be concerned about maintaining control over their lives.

ETHICS AND ELIGIBILITY

Mr. Brown knows that if he inquires long enough, he will discover some asset that disqualifies the client from eligibility for the program. It is remarkable that our health care system requires "spend-down" for long-term care eligibility but not for acute rescue interventions. However unfair this imbalance is, the fact remains that spend-down policies are widespread, and that society is reluctant to provide long-term care when familial resources remain available. Despite the moral ambiguity of spend-down, so long as it exists, it should be applied fairly. If property restrictions are to be challenged, this should be a matter of wide public debate and formal policy.

Mr. Brown does not want to know about his client's small savings account or insurance policy that might mean ineligibility and disqualification from the program. It is not his responsibility to actively delve into these financial matters. But if previously unrevealed resources are disclosed to him, he then has a duty to bring that to wider attention. Justice to those who truly abide by spend-down regulations requires this. Eligibility must be based consistently on genuine need.

Mr. Brown is concerned with a client who owns a $10,000 to $15,000 property, and refuses to sell it. In my view, Mr. Brown should enforce the eligibility rules, regardless of how adamant the client is about leaving the property to his church. There is literally no end to the kinds of hopes and desires that people have when it comes to leaving properties to favored organization and individuals. Exceptions imperil the entire system.

Again, I have serious reservations about spend-down policies. When an individual needs acute life-saving care, we do not require that his or her family spend down nearly all assets to become eligible for support. I accept the notion that families have a significant financial responsibility to provide long-term care, but the eligibility standards, though not as devastating in some states as they once were, are still too demanding. Few articulate the resource asymmetry between acute and long-term care better than Daniel Callahan (1990), however much his idea of age-based cutoffs of life-saving care can be scrutinized (Binstock and Post, 1991).

WAITING LISTS

A just health care system would balance support for acute and long-term care. When medical technology saves lives, it is imperative that something be done to make those lives livable. The success of modern medicine adds years of life to those who, in a previous time, would have died. Accident victims with spinal cord injuries are saved now for lives of sometimes total dependency on others. Imperiled neonates are saved as well, often a permanent burden on their families. Our health care system must deal with the consequences of rescue and acute care interventions by enhancing the quality of life for those whose lives have been lengthened.

Compared with other societies, ours does not have the necessary balance between acute- and long-term care. Survivors and their families may suffer extreme hardships. In the meanwhile, countless futile and highly expensive technologies are applied to patients in hospitals, and resources are routinely wasted.

The very fact that there are waiting lists for case management is unjust. Waiting lists do exist, testimony to a skewed health care system that has been inattentive to the broad spectrum of needs from prevention to long-term care. So long as such lists plague clients and case managers, some attention to the urgency of client need should be given, coupled with a first-come, first-serve factor.

Queuing up, with special consideration for cases of severe immediate need, would be reasonable, at least theoretically. It may be the case that in practice, distinguishing between degrees of urgency is very complicated and time-consuming. Nevertheless, some lines between urgent and less pressing cases can be sketched out. The other possibility would be to ration whatever resources are available evenly to all those clients in need, so that a minimal universal coverage would be the norm. My preference is for queuing up, partly because then more pressure can be placed on government to provide for those who still await needed intervention. There is a sense in which a minimal but universal approach, because it covers everyone somewhat, might be interpreted to mean that enough resources are available. Politically and strategically, it is better to have a line of people without any assistance, because they are witnesses to injustices that must then be corrected. If everyone gets some minimal intervention, injustice is obscured.

REFERENCES

Binstock, R. H., & Post, S. G. (1991). *Too old for health care? Controversies in medicine, law, economics, and ethics*. Baltimore: Johns Hopkins University Press.

Brody, E. M. (1990). *Women in the middle: Their parent-care years*. New York: Springer.

Callahan, D. (1990). *What kind of life: The limits of medical progress*. New York: Simon & Schuster.

Douglas, A. (1979). *The feminization of American culture*. New York: Avon.

Post, S. G. (1990). Women and elderly parents: Moral controversy in an aging society. *Hypatia: A Journal of Feminist Philosophy, 5,* 83–89.

Rawls, J. (1971). *A theory of justice*. Cambridge, MA: Harvard University Press.

VIEW FROM THE FIELD

Perspective From Wisconsin

■

Donna McDowell

RESOURCE ALLOCATION

By definition, situations that require a case manager should be complex, reflect great need for services, and have a well-defined target population and meet a uniform eligibility screen (reflecting need). Once consumers are accepted in the program, their needs should be met in a manner they find acceptable. Case managers do not have a responsibility to judge who is deserving. The subsequent points follow from this:

- We shouldn't short-change one client to add another to the roll. (We don't allow nursing homes to exceed their licensed capacity or double-bunk; we only do that in prisons.)
- Case managers who underserve clients artificially lower the "average cost" used to calculate budgets for state programs, thus perpetuating resource limitations.
- Meeting individual preferences may take more planning but doesn't have to cost more (e.g., Mr. Brown could use his 4 hours of paid home care at either end of the day to ease the niece's schedule. A paid informal provider might replace an agency service. Is the niece paid? Why not?).
- Family care saves money in the long-term care system. Investing in caregiver relief service helps keep the family care intact.
- Have other family members or volunteers been solicited to provide weekend respite, make reassuring telephone calls, do shopping, laundry, bills? The nature of family relations makes some ties stronger, but others can play a suitable role.
- Is day care and its related transport too expensive? Would the money be better spent adding hours of home care to relieve the niece?

AGENCIES' RESPONSIBILITIES AND RIGHTS

Modern business is investing in quality which delights the customer. In business, quality pays. Agencies can be expected to operate in a competitive environment. Therefore, the following seem reasonable:

- As purchaser, the case manager can reward quality with referrals.
- Rules that restrict freedom of choice endanger quality.
- Providers should have to adapt to needs of the customer, not the reverse.

ELIGIBILITY AND SPEND-DOWN

Rules are intended to ensure equity. Rules defining eligibility or ability to pay should be applied equitably. Having said this, it should also be noted that client values regarding the dignity of owning assets reflect societal values (at least for that community or cohort). The aspirations of heirs should have no weight in enforcing spend-down, but there should be some opportunity for clients to be able to reward relatives for services rendered in order to reduce an unbearable sense of obligation. These values are continually in conflict in long-term care.

- Case managers should apply rules fairly without assuming the role of auditors. (Nor should they be held accountable if auditors find what they missed.) Case management does not incorporate the functions of quality control for welfare systems.
- Case managers can assist a client to spend-down legally by recommending expenditures acceptable to the client, such as home improvements or modifications or purchase of appliances or adaptive equipment.
- Case managers can encourage clients to spend-down by paying for care and thereby extending their period of self-sufficiency.
- Mr. Brown could ask the church to encourage the client to look after his own needs (if this doesn't breach confidentially) and devise an alternate way he can help the church as a volunteer.

HOW MUCH IS TOO MUCH?

Client preferences reflect values and life-style choices. These values are more often satisfied by *how* the service is delivered (quality) rather than how much (quantity) is given. A case manager must become informed about the time, frequency, and manner of service preferred. These arrangements have to be negotiated with providers. Family members who give care should be consulted carefully about what they enjoy doing, when and how often. Negotiating limits on the scope, duration, and type of family service can accommodate the needs of the caregiver and the strength of their relationship to the consumer. The importance of family in social interaction, companionship, and sustaining a family role for the consumer should be valued as highly in a care plan as the instrumental tasks they could perform.

- Many older persons are almost pathologically grateful and will not express preferences for different service configurations.
- Many older persons will prefer family caregivers to strangers. In our culture, we can rarely take for granted family care from anyone but a spouse. And spouses of the same age will be fragile. Plans should then be built to facilitate family care, focusing on supporting the caregiver as a central purpose.

WAITING LISTS

Management of waiting lists is a responsibility of the case-management *agency*. Case managers should have input into policies for waiting lists, but not make them on a case-by-case basis. Advocacy groups should be kept apprised of waiting lists and legislators should have the same information.

- All customers in the queue should be assessed and advised of their options as well as the projected waiting time.
- Provisions should be made for *short-term* nursing home placements, if needed, without jeopardizing wait list status.
- Referrals should be made to any available services (e.g., meals, volunteer visitors) without jeopardizing wait list status.
- Agency (or government policies) can and should establish priorities beyond first-come, first-served. Categories of need can be established, and "first-come" rules apply within such categories. For example,

  Terminally ill (elderly, those with AIDS)
  Developmentally disabled children of frail aging parents
  Infirmity or loss of caregiver
  Repeated mental health crises resulting in costly hospitalizations
  Proportional groupings of young and old disabled
  Length of time on wait list

Case managers need to view the elements of quality in their work as providing the best, most cost-effective service tailored to satisfy the needs of *each* customer without preference or prejudice. Supervisors and managers need to support that role by assuming the harder tasks of making policies about rationing and equity. Training and supervision of case managers should reflect the reality that case managers will feel judgmental about who gets too much or too little but the real measure of their performance is meeting objective need in a manner that satisfies the preferences of the customer.

EDITORS' QUESTIONS FOR FURTHER DISCUSSION

■

1. To what extent should we require care plans that involve similar hours for similar levels of disability? Should client fastidiousness or previous life-style be considered in making plans more or less parsimonious?
2. What requirements are imposed by equity considerations for family members? Under what circumstances should one client's family get off the hook when another has to give care? Because of their geographical proximity? Their willingness? Their capability? Their life-styles and opportunity costs?
3. How much can a family member reasonably be expected to do? Does the type of relationship—e.g., spouse, offspring, other relative—make a difference, or does willingness count for all? Is the case manager ever morally obliged to rescue a family member even though costs to the program will increase?
4. What constitutes appropriate fairness to agencies and providers? Should this be the case manager's concern?
5. What would be a fair way of adding new clients? Are waiting list policies intrinsically fair? Is a first-come, first-served policy fair? Should property restrictions be challenged?
6. How is a case manager to balance multiple fairness claims?

Chapter 14

CONCLUSION: Toward an Ethic of Case Management

Rosalie A. Kane, Arthur L. Caplan, and Cheryl King Thomas

Case management may seem an unlikely subject in search of an ethic. It is hardly a household word—many health and human services professionals have only the dimmest idea that case managers exist and that their decisions could influence the well-being of their patients or clients. Older persons with disabilities are even less likely to know about case managers. The ethical struggles of physicians, nurses, and even social workers may capture the public imagination from time to time, whereas case management sounds bureaucratic, dull, and irrelevant.

Case management is, in fact, under development. It is an emerging occupation. Many of its methods and techniques are unsettled or in contention. It is practiced by people who may owe allegiances to a variety of disciplines—social work, nursing, and others (many of which have codes of ethics of their own), and it is also practiced by college graduates with "social worker" or "case manager" in their job titles, but no formal professional affiliations. By and large, case managers work for agencies, and the administrative rules of those agencies may enhance or seriously limit the case managers' ability to respect autonomy, to be beneficent, and to be just. Thus the ethics of case managers are inextricably linked to the ethical premises of the agencies through which they practice.

Perhaps it would be prudent to let the ethics of case management wait until the field itself has become more settled into orthodoxy. But case management is such a widespread function in long-term care programs, and case managers contend with so many difficult problems with such far-reaching implications for the people they serve that the ethics considerations cannot await the codification of the practice. Right now, case managers are entrusted to make important decisions with and for frail elderly and disabled persons. They struggle with all the predictable problems of balancing beneficence and respect for autonomy, as well as the multiple interests of clients and family members. Indeed, better charting of the ethics territory may provide guidance for how the field itself is defined and shaped.

ECOLOGY OF CASE MANAGEMENT

This much we do know. Case managers have a great deal to say about the care that functionally disabled older people receive. They are paid (though in many cases hardly handsomely) to make judgments about the care needs of their fellow human beings, and to help them—their clients—arrange for needed services. They are expected to determine when their clients can safely live in the community, usually always in the context of knowing that only a finite pool of resources are available to spend on all clients. They are expected to respect clients' preferences and rights to autonomy all the while, unless, of course, the client is incapable of decision making. And the case manager is also expected to be able to discern when the client is or is not capable of such decision making. These are important, almost awesome responsibilities, and there is much evidence that many case managers take them seriously.

We also know that the everyday stuff of a case manager's life involves working with many clients whose heavy needs for care seem to make a mockery of the slender resources the case manager can muster. Such clients may cling, nonetheless, to the familiarity and comfort of their homes and resist the case manager's views that they would be safer elsewhere. Case managers perpetually worry about risks to the health and well-being of their frail clients. These concerns are exacerbated if, as is frequently the case, the client's cognitive capacities are waning, fluctuating, or very impaired.

Case management decisions often include multiple parties. We know that case management entails work with families, mostly (though not always) benevolent, caring, and caregiving families. Case managers must balance competing views within families about what is best for elderly or disabled relatives, sometimes dealing with discrepant views of the client and the family caregivers. And because the unpaid labor of family members is an implicit and often explicit part of most plans for care at home, families surely have legitimate interests in the decisions that implicate them. But when that interest gets translated into a veto power over risks the client may want to assume, case managers become troubled and uncertain how to proceed.

We know also that the business of case managers frequently involves the behind-the-scenes interests of the various care providers who are contracted to assist the client or who are somehow involved in the case. For example, the case manager typically purchases service from home care agencies and monitors its quality, and sometimes disputes arise about the amount and type of service ordered. Sometimes clients object to the providers chosen by the case manager. Case managers are conscious of their power to alter the census and therefore the fate of the various agencies in the community by the way they make referrals or purchase care. Struggling to be simultaneously fair to the providers, respectful of their clients' preferences, and mindful of their clients' best interests, case managers ask themselves whether they have the right to make specific referrals and recommendations, and whether they have the right to talk clients out of using a particular agency, or even a particular physician.

Finally, we know that case managers' decisions are often less clearcut than those made by physicians about medical treatments. Similarly, the decisions and choices of their clients are more diffuse and less easy to isolate than the decisions about a particular course of action or treatment. Thus, the work of the case manager requires steady attention.

We know that at least some of the business of case managers is conducted in the glare of public attention. When an eccentric person's physical dependencies puts him or her in public view; or when a person *becomes* eccentric and troublesome because of age-related impairments; or when the stereotypical neglected home makes neighbors fear for their own health or property values, the public claims a stake in what case managers decide. Furthermore, the case manager who watches and worries rather than sets in motion competency hearings and relocation may be viewed as neglectful by well-intentioned observers. Case managers and their employers worry that events may even occasionally bear out the worst predictions of onlookers. The single untoward incident—a fire, an injury to a third party—could bring down an official inquiry and discredit the program.

In modern hospitals, for better or worse, decision makers have layers of protection—risk managers, ethicists, internal and external quality assurance groups, a body of case law, and the comfort afforded by "team" decision making. Not so case managers. For the most part, they make decisions alone, often without time for reflection. The volume and routine nature of their work—doing assessments, making care plans, authorizing services, doing reassessments—partly masks the momentous nature of the results to the people they serve. But not completely. The study results presented in chapter 2 and the case examples derived from that study, which are explored in the subsequent chapters, attest that many case managers are vitally concerned about the ethical ramifications of their work, which so shapes the last years of many older people. We can hardly justify putting the ethics of case-managed long-term care on the back-burner while we continue to refine exquisitely the ethics of the last days and hours of life.

MORAL LEGITIMACY OF CASE MANAGEMENT

First, a fundamental question could be raised: Is case management itself a legitimate enterprise that is right and proper? This requires consideration of its goals, its authority, its inherent paternalism, and the question of whether case management is a poor second to some better approach to care arrangements.

Some skeptics question the authority by which case managers take part in decisions about how much care an individual needs, or whether an individual can be cared for safely at home within available resources. Who, they ask, are these people called case managers, and what gives them the right to be involved in the case? Spokespersons for some disabled persons reinforce this position by questioning whether a case manager's assessment is ever a proper basis for allocating services. How, they ask, can anyone properly know how much and what kind of help a person needs to conduct his or her life? Only the person most concerned could make that determination. Ethicists who are wedded to the principle of respect for autonomy may find that argument strikes an answering cord.

Others suggest that the development of case management is a failure of human services rather than a higher stage in their evolution. For example, case management could be construed as an expedient to cover up for a shoddy and underfunded system of care. In that view, if affordable, high-quality services were available and easily accessible, much of the need for case management would disappear.

These questions can be approached in an orderly fashion, but they each need work. First, the authority for case management is derived from statutes and their accompanying regulations that make long-term care services at home available to persons with functional impairments. The eligibility for and scope of these services vary from state to state, but almost every state has some such programs in place. Case managers are responsible for screening applicants to make sure that they fall within the targeted eligibility group and for allocating services according to need. Also, given that the programs work within budgets, case managers control the use of the resources, trying to spread them so that they do the most good. Within such programs, one could argue that justice requires some sort of case-management function. Furthermore, even if we went to the systems level to consider the ethics of case-managed programs, we would be hard-put to argue the justice of a open-ended entitlement to long-term care services.

It follows that the arguments against the inherent paternalism of a case manager's assessment are also ill founded. If people wish to avail themselves of a public or publicly subsidized benefit, they surely also should accept the intrusiveness of some scrutiny into their relative need for that benefit. Thus, there are no grounds for rejecting a case manager's assessment and determination of need out of hand. However, it is highly appropriate for disabled people of all ages and citizens at large to ask second-order questions about the role and premises of case management. For example, is the case manager's assessment sensitive to real needs of the disabled person? To what extent should the case manager be able to dictate how and where the service resources are used for a person who has been assessed as eligible for the assistance? Should people have the option of managing their own case in the sense of distributing the fixed sum of money made available to help them compensate for their functional impairments? What amount of money— which should, after all, be used to pay for help for people with functional impairments, should be syphoned off to pay case managers for checking on the quality of the ongoing care and the safety of the client? Should those who arguably do not need such surveillance get more funds for services themselves? These kinds of questions are fair game, and ethical examination of case-management programs should help determine answers.

What about the notion that case management represents a failure of service systems to present intelligible, accessible, and visible programs that potential users can find and afford? There is some merit to this argument but not enough to discredit case management as a function. It seems obvious that the more readily services are available, the less hard case managers will need to work to patch together a plan. But case managers work in arenas where the needs are complex and interacting;

where some technical assessment and continued diagnosis is required to sort them out; where the services required cross over into jurisdictions like acute care, primary care, and mental health. The skilled assessment of the case manager is truly required, at least some of the time. Then, too, case managers work with and on behalf of persons who cannot manage their own case—perhaps because they are very sick, because they have communication and sensory impairment, or because they have cognitive impairments. These deficits may be temporary or permanent. Some might offer the rejoinder that it is up to families to manage the case when the disabled person cannot. However, as the cases in this book demonstrate, family members are often divided among themselves and from the client in determining what should be done, and they too may be bereft of the information and technical skills needed to sort things out.

Finally, a word about the goals of case management. Although it is conventional to begin any inquiry by considering goals, it somehow is clearer to think of the goals of case management—itself a rather abstract notion—in relation to the authority for the enterprise and the kinds of work case managers do. Given that case management is used to allocate services, the goals of case management can be viewed on an individual level and a systems level, and considerable variation is possible in both spheres. For example, at the individual level, the case manager's goal could be to postpone or avoid admissions to nursing homes, to enhance clients' physical functioning, to provide relief and support for family members, or, more expansively, to enhance social involvement and emotional well-being. The case-management program may or may not also have an explicit goal of maximizing autonomy and choice for functionally impaired older people. At the system level, the goal could be to provide in-home service equitably to those in need; to reduce public expenditures on nursing home care or other services; more ambitiously, to use the purchasing power to improve the quality and responsiveness of available services in the community; or, similarly, to reduce the unit prices of services and thus increase their availability to clients. There may or may not also be a goal that substantial volunteered family labor continue in the care of the frail elderly. None of these goals are improper on the face of it; each could be debated for their ethical nuances.

In practice, case-management programs often promulgate multiple, even conflicting goals (For example, a program may aspire to promote maximum physical, mental, and social well-being of clients while also keeping clients out of nursing homes and saving money for the state). The programs from which our sample cases were derived had varying objectives and varied also in the degree to which the goals were explicit.

Yet a clear-eyed understanding of program goals and some sense of priorities among them is surely a prerequisite for the ethical conduct of case management. Otherwise case managers and clients alike will have confused expectations.

ETHICAL THEMES IN CASE MANAGEMENT

Combination of Advocacy and Gatekeeping

We argue that there is nothing intrinsically wrong with case management in the moral sense, and, in fact, it is a moral endeavor. Questions can be raised, however, about the ethical premises in a role that combines advocacy for a client and gatekeeping of resources. Much of the anguish of case managers revolves around reconciling these roles.

As advocates, case managers are expected to get to perform a multidimensional assessment, to develop an informed understanding about the kinds of services the client needs and prefers, to suggest a package of services that meets those needs and preferences, to help clients and family members accept the intrusiveness of services in their homes, and to alleviate any fears that becoming a case-management or home care client means that bureaucrats will henceforth judge their adequacy to live at home. To do so adequately, they must come to know their clients intimately and win their trust.

As gatekeepers, case managers may be expected to be parsimonious, to offer no more service than is minimally needed, to rely on volunteered family care whenever possible (even if this is not ideally what either client or family member prefers), to make recommendations for alternative living situations when a care plan at home becomes prohibitively expensive, and to recommend reductions in service if the client's functioning improves commensurately. Arguably, the case manager as gatekeeper is an advocate for a whole community of disabled and elderly persons, and attempts to spread out the resources.

Perhaps calling the case manager an advocate obscures the fact that advocacy occurs within the limits of the gatekeeping and resource-allocating roles. Perhaps, too, there if clients rely on case managers for information and advice and case managers fail to disclose the full range of services for which they might be eligible. Nancy Dubler, an attorney and ethicist, has argued that one can never be a true advocate as a program official whose budget cannot be balanced unless some people forego services to which they are theoretically entitled. For example, eligibility for services under most long-term care statutes is based strictly on the measurable functional impairment of the disabled person, but programs stretch their funds as far as they do only because they rely on available family members to keep on providing large amounts of care.

Informed Consent

We are optimistic that advocacy and resource allocation can be united in the same person and program without violation of ethical precepts, though the prerequisites for this accomplishment may be difficult to reach. In fact, it requires exquisite attention to informed consent.

Clients and family members must understand what case management is, the constraints under which the programs operate, and the limits to the advice that is offered. They must also be informed about their rights to reject the recommendations of case managers, along with the implications of such rejection. (In some programs, all services may be withdrawn if the client persists in what the case manager considers a risky course, whereas in others this will not be the case.)

Informed consent in case management also extends to an explanation about the kinds of questions that the assessment entails, and the way the information will be used. Clients also need to understand the nature of the case manager's ongoing role, and his or her relationship to the providers of service. Thus, the client will know whether he or she can alter the details of the care plan and whether requests should be directed to the providers or the case managers. Clients must know how the case manager construes the relationship with family members. For example, will the case manager keep some matters confidential from family members at the client's request? Is the program predicated on an expectation that the family will be involved with the client's care? Finally, clients should know whether case managers have agreements with particular providers of care, and what their real choices are for subsidized care from care providers of the same or different types.

It is our impression that informed consent processes have not been well thought out in case management. The very act of raising the questions in the previous paragraph surfaces issues that ethicists could systematically explore.

Privacy and Confidentiality

A series of issues about confidentiality and privacy are related to the informed consent issues, but should be considered independently. Informed consent makes clear to the client how information will be used and when privacy will be protected, but the moral foundation for these arrangements is a prior consideration.

Case managers collect systematic, at times voluminous, information about their clients. They establish a record of the assessment, which is the basis for the services that the clients receive. When they arrange services, they may share that information formally or informally with service providers. Typically, the clients sign a blanket permission that the information collected can be shared within the hierarchy of the case management agency and with service providers. Yet, is such widespread sharing of information necessary and proper? This question is particularly apt when the case manager's assessment ranges broadly to encompass the client's whole biography.

The rhetoric about confidentiality often outstrips the reality. To make an analogy, despite widespread commitment to notions of medical confidentiality, medical records in hospitals are hardly confidential any longer. The clinical teams are too large and diffuse to truly restrict the flow of information. Third-party payers have a stake in learning information about the patient. So too, perhaps, with case management. Indeed, if confidentiality is illusory, it might be more useful to set a high standard for respect for privacy and work to make that operational rather than perpetuate an allusion that anything uttered to the case manager is confidential in the strictest sense of the word.

Client Choice

The very term *case management* gives discomfort. Nobody wants to be a "case," and nobody wants to be managed. Even if the softer term, *care coordination*, is substituted, the core question remains: How much decision-making prerogatives should case managers have on the details of the care plan? To what extent does the case manager have an obligation to respect the choices of the client? What if the client might choose more, less, or different care details than the case manager considers optimal? What if the client's choices cost more money, yet still are in the range that the program considers permissible?

Because long-term care plans can be all-encompassing and intrusive, separations between the care and the life-style the care enables are difficult to make. Thus, managing or coordinating the client's care could glide into managing the client's life. Case mangers tend to have large case loads and easily drift into standard procedures to translate needs for service into care packages. Even with excellent intentions to respect client autonomy and a program that allows them flexibility, they may fail to describe to the client the wide array of options that could be used to address the functional impairment. Clients, in turn, might be un-aware of the many interchangeable ways to meet their needs. Even when clients sign off on care plans, they may be unaware of the range of options and have no real input into the plan.

Many of our cases involved the paradoxical preference of the clients for *less* help than the case manager thought would be most beneficial. Although insurance companies and governments worry about the "mor-al hazard" of covering attractive home-based long-term care services, clients who are entitled to these services often need to be cajoled into accepting them. There seems to be a self-protective instinct among many clients that "less is more" when it comes to home care. Clients may also resist specific parts of the plan—such as seeing a doctor, going to a day care center, or undergoing alcohol treatment. Deliberation is needed about the extent to which clients should be free to reject parts of a care plan.

What about client choice of case manager? In that respect, case man-agers have been viewed more like school teachers or hospital nurses than physicians, psychotherapists, or attorneys. In theory, people choose the latter and terminate relationships that are unsatisfactory, whereas the teacher and nurse come with their organizations and ordi-narily the preference of the student or patient is irrelevant. To the extent that the case manager and clients are expected to form a close relation-ship of trust, one might wish to structure some way that the client could choose a compatible case manager, or at least provide an opportunity for the client to request a change of case manager. Conversely, case manag-ers exercising professional judgment and working within program rules are bound to make decisions from time to time that displease the clients. Case assignments are distributed according to some logic (geography or rotation, perhaps) and too much client choice would play havoc with efficiency of case management. Moreover, clients would ordinarily have no basis on which to exercise their original choice. Still, some-thing seems amiss in a program that respects consumer choice (in-cluding choice of the caregivers who enter their homes), if no provision is made for choice regarding the case manager who puts it all into motion.

Termination of Treatment

Termination of treatment considerations are an ethics staple for physi-cians, who must function with a clear idea of when a relationship with a patient may be ended without constituting abandonment. In case man-agement, it is not at all clear what should constitute the end point of the relationship. Indeed, programs now vary in their operating practices. In some programs, case managers cease their involvement with the client when the client no longer receives services purchased by the plan, in others when the client enters a nursing home, and in others, only with the client's death. Some case managers continue their relationship of advice, support, and advocacy when no services are currently being received, either because they are no longer necessary or because they are not available, the latter either because of general lack of services or lack of services in a form acceptable to the client.

Again, to the extent that the relationship includes advocacy, expert advice, and support, and assuming that the client is satisfied with the case manager, one could argue that withdrawal of that support is unjustified merely because of a failure to arrive at an adequate, mutually satisfactory plan. However, case managers and their supervisors may believe that continuation of case management makes them complicit in an inadequate or unsafe plan. The average long-term care client is very old, has multiple impairments, and has a shaky family support system. Her life will be full of more than the average uncertainty and risk. With or without case management, whether she stays at home or enters a nursing home, whether her care plan is lavish or meager, she is likely to be within a few years of death, and her health could at any time take a turn for the worse. The case manager, along with the client, must be able to live with the risks and uncertainties that the client chooses. It may be easier for case managers to stand by their cases despite less than perfect care plans if they recall that the usual alternative—entering a nursing home—is hardly risk free. It is just that the case manager is unlikely to know the end of the story if termination is automatic when the client enters a nursing home.

VIRTUES OF CASE MANAGERS

Another way of thinking about ethics and case management is to consider what constitutes virtue in a case manager. From the cases and commentaries in this book, a tentative list of virtues of case managers emerges.

The case manager should be creative and imaginative. This is the characteristic that allows the virtuous case manager to make the extra effort to enhance the client's autonomy and preferences. To do so often requires imaginative exploration of new ways to meet a need. Creativity is perhaps the virtue that can most often be inferred from the case material.

The case manager should be flexible. This virtue is a corollary to creativity. The case manager must be ready to vary his or her approach, her plans, and even the use of his or her own time, if he or she is truly individualizing the cases.

The case manager should be tolerant and open-minded. Older people are as varied as human kind itself—only more so. (It is an axiom of gerontology that variability increases with age.) Only the tolerant case manager can hope to enter into the experience and goals of the wide range of clients who he or she may encounter.

The case manager should be persistent. This trait of perseverance is important not only because the good case manager endeavors to reach a satisfactory plan one way or another, trying first one approach and then an alternative. It also may be important as a characteristic that allows the case manager to remain involved in a case even when it seems to be going downhill, even when there is little to do but watch and wait for the next crisis.

The case manager should be available. Case managers need to be physically and emotionally accessible to their clients. At times of crisis or potential change—for example, when the client has entered a hospital— the client should be able to find the virtuous case manager.

The case manager should be fair. This includes procedural fairness but is not limited to narrow rule following. The case manager should appreciate the spirit as well as the letter of the law.

The case manager should be trustworthy. The virtuous case manager recognizes that he or she is privy to personal details of the client's life and situation, and that such a trust cannot be treated casually.

The case manager looks critically at the case-management program. Virtuous case managers notice when program rules impede rather than foster the well-being or autonomy of clients. They notice if, case after case, the kinds of services most desired are the ones the program excludes from payment. Case managers should be committed to improving the program over time and be observant about the steps to be taken.

The case manager should be competent. Even though case management is an emerging field, there is usually a technology in place. Case managers can choose to take their techniques such as assessment, care planning, and monitoring of services seriously, to learn how to do them well, and to hone their skills as case managers. This requires learning how to ask awkward questions comfortably, learning how to cost out a care plan, learning how to negotiate with families, learning in detail about the type and quality of services provided by agencies in the community, and learning specifically how to get feedback on the adequacy of a worker in the home. If the case manager skips questions on the assessment form rather than learn how to ask them; if the case manager omits inquiring about the values and preferences of the client; if the case manager's plans do not follow from the particulars of a client's needs; if the case manager's monitoring is haphazard or limited to receiving complaints—then the case manager cannot be said to be performing competently.

Each of the proposed virtues, of course, has its organizational counterpart. If the case manager is to be creative, flexible, tolerant, persistent, available, fair, trustworthy, competent, and self-critical, the organization must foster these qualities through its training, its expectations, its procedures, and its reward structure.

NEXT STEPS

This consideration of case management ethics was meant to be a beginning. We consider it important in its own right, simply because case management is occurring, and problems about what case managers should do and what their clients should, therefore, expect have surfaced from that practice.

The inquiry is important also because case-management practice in long-term care brings into sharper relief issues that have not been in the forefront of bioethics. These include issues of familial responsibility (which could feasibly come up in the acute care sector but tend not to); issues of fairness across gender (when most of the clients and case managers are women but the authority figures in the legal system are men); ethics in the roles of paraprofessional in-home workers, whose jobs combine heavy responsibility and minimal authority; and even the ethical issues inherent in a system of long-term care that revolves around a nursing home that is structured so as to be abhorrent to those who might need to use it. Case-management programs are in a position to bear witness to these issues, to flesh them out with case examples, and to add to the agenda of bioethics in a substantial way.

There is much to be done, and the time-honored tools are available for doing it. Development of ethics committees would be useful. Development, refinement, and evaluation of structures to make case management programs as protective of clients and as fair as possible is also necessary including informed consent procedures and appeals processes. Elaboration of the science and art of case management is also needed including ways to assess adequately the values and preferences of the clients being served. Ethicists as well as health and social service professionals need to pay attention to this burgeoning area, and to consider whether the principles that have seemed to help in solving problems in the acute care area need modification in light of what case managers tell us.

The ethical challenge of case management is summed up by the many paradoxes of the enterprise. Case managers must perform a routine function reliably yet make fine distinctions. They must be consistent yet flexible. They are advocates and gatekeepers both. They work within a system of services, yet must chronicle its limitations and strive for improvements. They take on responsibility for a client's well-being, yet must accept that they cannot protect the client from risks. It is little wonder that case managers appreciate the ethical tensions in their work. We hope that articulating the problems is a step toward addressing them well.

CONTRIBUTORS

Adrienne Asch, PhD, served as a Senior Human Rights Specialist at the New York State Division of Human Rights and as Associate in Social Science and Policy with the New Jersey Bioethics Commission. She holds a degree in social work, and received her doctorate in social psychology from Columbia University in 1992. She is on the faculty of the Boston University School of Social Work and the Boston University program in Law, Medicine, and Ethics.

Baruch Brody, PhD, is the Leon Jaworski Professor of Biomedical Ethics and the Director of the Center for Ethics, Medicine, and Public Issues at the Baylor College of Medicine. He is also a Professor of Philosophy at Rice University and an Adjunct Research Fellow at the Institute of Religion. His most recent book, published by Oxford University Press, is *Life and Death Decision Making*.

Richard Browdie, MBA, is Deputy Secretary with the Pennsylvania Department of Aging. He has administered protective services and community-based long-term care services at the local and state level since 1975.

Sean Browne is Coordinator of Eldercare Services with the Oklahoma State Department of Health.

Arthur L. Caplan, PhD, is the Director of the Center for Biomedical Ethics at the University of Minnesota, where he is also a Professor of Philosophy and a Professor of Surgery. Among his recent books: *If I Were A Rich Man Could I Buy A Pancreas and Other Essays on the Ethics of Health Care* (Indiana University Press), *When Medicine Went Mad: Bioethics and the Holocaust* (Humana), and *Everyday Ethics: Resolving Dilemmas in Nursing Home Life* (Springer), which he co-edited with Rosalie A. Kane.

Bart J. Collopy, PhD, is Associate for Ethical Studies at the Third Age Gerontology Center and Associate Professor in the Humanities Division, Fordham University at Lincoln Center. His recent writing has focused on such topics as autonomy in long term care, the ethics of using restraints, and the moral quandaries of home care. In 1990 he co-edited, with Connie Zuckerman and Nancy Dubler, *Home Health Care Options* (Plenum Press).

Susan L. Dietsche, MSW, is Assistant Administrator with the Oregon Senior and Disabled Services Division. She received her MSW from Portland State University. A specialist in long-term-care-delivery systems, she has consulted and made numerous presentations on aspects of the "Oregon Systems" and long-term care.

Rebecca Dresser, JD, is a Professor in the School of Law and the Center for Biomedical Ethics in the School of Medicine at Case Western Reserve University. She has been teaching medical ethics and law since 1983. She has written and lectured extensively on issues raised by advance treatment directives and on the appropriate standards to govern treatment for incompetent patients.

Rebecca Elon, MD, MPH, joined the faculty of the Division of Geriatric Medicine at the Francis Scott Key Medical Center, Johns Hopkins University School of Medicine, as an Assistant Professor in 1991. She trained in internal medicine and geriatrics at Baylor College of Medicine in Houston, Texas, and completed her studies in public health at the University of Texas Health Science Center in Houston. She is a participant in the Kellogg National Fellowship Program.

Amitai Etzioni, PhD, is the first University Professor of The George Washington University. During 1987–1989, he was the Thomas Henry Carroll Ford Foundation Professor at the Harvard Business School. He was Senior Adviser in the White House during 1979–1980, and guest scholar at the Brookings Institution during 1978–1979. For 20 years (1958–1978) he was Professor of Sociology at Columbia University. He was the founding president of the international Society for the Advancement of Socio-Economics. He is the editor of *The Responsive Community* and the author of fourteen books, including *The Moral Dimension: Toward a New Economics*.

Mary Lou Hartland, MSW, is Intergenerational Coordinator with the Delaware Division on Aging. She has been the Statewide Administrator for the Case Management Program that also encompassed home health care contracts and Adult Foster Care.

Brian Hofland, PhD, is Vice President of the Retirement Research Foundation in Chicago, Illinois. In this capacity, he developed and managed a $2 million, five-year special interdisciplinary initiative examining the legal, ethical, and practical issues involved in enhancing the autonomy of older adults in long-term care. He was guest editor of a recent issue of *Generations* entitled, "Autonomy and Long Term Care Practice."

Robert Hornyak is Assistant Director of the Aging/In-Home Services Section of the Indiana Division of Aging and Rehabilitative Services.

Rosalie A. Kane, DSW, is a professor in the Institute for Health Services Research at the University of Minnesota. Previously, she was a Senior Researcher at The Rand Corporation, and a faculty member at University of California at Los Angeles and the University of Utah. She conducts research and provides technical assistance on long-term care, with particular reference to quality of home care and nursing home care, long-term care system design and financing, case management, assessments, and values and ethics. With Arthur Caplan she edited the 1991 book, *Everyday Ethics: Resolving Dilemmas in Everyday Life*. She is the author of seven other books, including *Long-Term Care Principles, Programs, and Policies* (with Robert Kane), and numerous articles and reports. From 1989–1992 she was editor-in-chief of *The Gerontologist*.

Helen Q. Kivnick, PhD, received her PhD in psychology from the University of Michigan. Currently on the faculty of the University of Minnesota School of Social Work, she has previously held teaching and research positions at the University of Chicago, the University of California, Berkeley, and Northwestern University. Her research includes studies of grandparenthood, and collaborative studies of developmental issues in aging with Erik and Joan Erikson, which led to their 1989 book, *Vital Involvement in Old Age*. She is currently engaged in studying role models for successful aging and, more recently, successful aging of people needing and receiving long-term care.

Mary B. Mahowald, PhD, a philosopher who has been "doing" ethics in the clinical setting since 1982, is currently Professor in the Pritzker School of Medicine and the College, and Senior Scholar in the Center for Clinical Medical Ethics at the University of Chicago. Her most recent book, *Women and Children in Health Care: An Unequal Majority*, was published by Oxford University Press.

Donna McDowell, MSS, serves as Director of the Wisconsin Bureau on Aging, Department of Health and Social Services. She holds a Master's degree in social services from Bryn Mawr College Graduate School. Currently the President of the National Association of State Units on Aging (1991–93), she is a frequent public speaker and occasional consultant in the U.S., Australia, and the U. K.

Steven H. Miles, MD, is a practicing geriatrician in the Division of Geriatric Medicine, Hennepin County Medical Center, and an Associate Professor of Medicine in the University of Minnesota Medical School. He is an ethicist with the University of Minnesota Center for Biomedical Ethics. He is co-author of the 1989 book, *Protocols for Elective Use of Life-Sustaining Treatment*.

Robert L. Mollica, MSSS, EdD, is a Professional Staff Member at the National Academy for State Health Policy in Portland, Maine. He conducts health policy research and provides technical assistance to state health policy leaders on a range of issues that includes access and the uninsured, financing and systems reform, and long-term care. He was formerly the Assistant Secretary for Policy and Program Development at the Massachusetts Executive Office of Elder Affairs. His responsibilities included long-term care, housing, health, mental health, transportation, consumer information, and state and federal legislation. Prior to joining the Executive Office of Elder Affairs, he worked in the Massachusetts Lieutenant Governor's Office of Federal Relations.

Todd A. Monson, BSN, MPH, is Program Manager of the Hennepin County Community Health Department's Community-Based Long Term Care Programs in Minneapolis, Minnesota.

Patrick Murphy is Chief of the Case Management Services Branch of the California Department of Aging, Long-Term Care, and Aging Services Division.

Joan Dobrof Penrod, MSSW, MA, is a Research Fellow at the University of Minnesota School of Public Health, Institute for Health Services Research. She has Master's degrees in social work and in business. She was a medical social worker for six years before moving into research in long-term care.

Stephen G. Post, PhD, is Associate Professor of biomedical ethics in the School of Medicine at Case Western Reserve University, and a Senior Research Fellow of the Kennedy Institute of Ethics at Georgetown University. He is also Senior Faculty Associate with the Center on Aging and Health, Case Western Reserve University. He serves as Associate Editor for the revised edition of the *Encyclopedia of Bioethics* (1993, Macmillan, 5 vols.), and is Associate Editor for ethics of *Alzheimer Disease* and *Associated Disorders: An International Journal* (Raven Press). He is co-editor, with Robert H. Binstock, PhD, of *Too Old for Health Care?* (Johns Hopkins University Press, 1991).

Don C. Postema, PhD, is a Professor in the Department of Philosophy at Bethel College, St. Paul, Minnesota. He is also the Hospital Ethics Consultant at St. Paul-Ramsey Medical Center, St. Paul, Minnesota. He was a Visiting Scholar at the Center for Biomedical Ethics, University of Minnesota, during 1992. His current research and teaching interests are in bioethics (the role of medical futility in clinical decision-making and health care policy) and aesthetics (interpretation and meaning in art).

Kathleen E. Powderly, CNM, MSN, MPhil, is the Assistant Director of the Division of Humanities in Medicine at the State University of New York Health Science Center at Brooklyn. She is also an Assistant Professor of Nursing and Obstetrics and Gynecology at the Health Science Center. She is a Certified Nurse-Midwife and has Masters' degrees in nursing and sociomedical sciences. She is a Ph.D. candidate at Columbia University in sociomedical sciences and lectures widely in areas of clinical ethics.

Reinhard Priester, JD, is a Research Associate with the Center for Biomedical Ethics at the University of Minnesota. His recent research and writing has focused on the ethical foundations of the U.S. health care system.

Charles E. Reed is Assistant Secretary with the Aging and Adult Services Administration in the State of Washington.

Muriel B. Ryden, PhD, RN, FAAN, is a Professor at the University of Minnesota School of Nursing. Her research and teaching interests are in gerontology (behavioral problems in persons with dementia) and ethics (autonomy of residents in long-term care and end-of-life decisions).

Carol Tauer, PhD, is Professor of Philosophy at the College of St. Catherine in St. Paul, Minnesota. Her research and writing focus on public policy issues related to bioethics. She has recently published articles on HIV testing, *in vitro* fertilization and other reproductive techniques, fetal tissue transplantation and research, and the human genome project. Currently, she is working on areas of maternal-fetal conflict such as refusal of caesarean section, and drug or alcohol abuse during pregnancy.

Cheryl King Thomas, MA, is a community program specialist with the University of Minnesota School of Public Health, Institute for Health Services Research. She holds a Master's degree in organizational communication and has coordinated long-term care research projects in home care, values and ethics preferences, and case management.

Oliver J. Williams, PhD, MPH, MSW, is an Assistant Professor in the School of Social Work at the University of Minnesota. His research focuses include multicultural issues and access to social services by minority populations and domestic violence as it applies to minority populations.

Susan M. Wolf, JD, is a 1992–93 Fellow in the Program in Ethics and the Professions at Harvard University. Prior to that, she was the Associate for Law at The Hastings Center in Briarcliff Manor, New York. She has also taught law and medicine at New York University as an Adjunct Associate Professor of Law, has served on the ethics committee at Memorial Sloan-Kettering Cancer Center, and is a former member of the New York City AIDS Review Panel. She has published on a range of topics in biomedical ethics and law, including death and dying, reproductive technologies, AIDS, and the patient/physician relationship.

Index